KU-050-712

THE RISKS OF PASSIVE SMOKING

ROY J. SHEPHARD

W. SUSSEX INSTITUTE
OF
HIGHER EDUCATION
LIBRARY

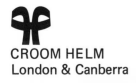
CROOM HELM
London & Canberra

© 1982 Roy J. Shephard
Croom Helm Ltd, 2-10 St John's Road, London SW11

British Library Cataloguing in Publication Data

Shephard, Roy J.
   The risks of passive smoking.
   1. Tobacco—Physiological effect
   I. Title
   613.8'5   RA1242.T6
   ISBN 0-7099-2334-1

Typeset by Leaper & Gard Ltd, Bristol
Printed and bound in Great Britain
by Billing and Sons Limited
Guildford, London, Oxford, Worcester

CONTENTS

To my family, who have granted me the
rich inheritance of a smoke-free home

INTRODUCTION

'. . . their roguish tobacco. It is good for nothing but to choke a man and fill him full of smoke and embers' — Ben Jonson, 1573–1637

'Herein is not only a great vanity, but a great contempt of God's good gifts, that the sweetness of man's breath, being a good gift of God, should be wilfully corrupted by this stinking smoke' — James I of England and VI of Scotland, 1566–1625

From the time of Ben Jonson's *Every Man out of his Humour* and the better known *A Counterblast to Tobacco* by James I, non-smokers have been conscious of the nuisance and annoyance created by an accumulation of tobacco smoke in enclosed spaces. Johann Wolfgang Von Goethe (1749–1832) captured the essence of their complaint: 'Smokers pollute the air far and wide and asphyxiate every respectable individual who cannot smoke in self-defence. Who can enter the room of a smoker without feeling nausea?'

The health hazards arising from such air pollution have been less clearly established. Cynics have held that the principal risk lay in the strength of tobacco addiction, and resultant confrontations between smokers and non-smokers. During the last few years, at least one commercial aircraft has been forced to make an emergency landing because of a fracas provoked by passengers who insisted upon smoking in a non-smoking section of the plane. The present author also had his glasses ground into his face (luckily without any permanent loss of vision), for the offence of advising a passenger that smoking was not permitted on a train. Nevertheless, the last two or three years have also brought powerful new evidence of the risks to health occasioned by unwanted exposure to cigarette smoke, or 'passive smoking' as it is popularly termed. Acute exposures to smoke-filled rooms have reduced the effort tolerance of patients with angina pectoris; chronic exposure to smoke-polluted air has apparently caused respiratory disease in young children and lung cancer in adults; while placental transfer of tobacco products has led smoking mothers to bear premature, underweight infants with continuing abnormalities of growth and development.

The fetus has no method of protesting the contamination of placental blood, other than a few well-aimed kicks, and the newborn child likewise can do little to dodge the nicotine-stained hand that rocks the cradle. In a modern, well-insulated home, even the spouse of an addict has little escape from accumulating smoke. The situation in public buildings, offices and vehicles has been more ambiguous, with cigarette manufacturers claiming that adequate protection of the non-smoker occupants could be ensured by a high ventilation rate. The energy crisis has necessitated an urgent re-examination of this belief. Buildings are being made evermore air-tight, to conserve heat in winter and refrigeration in summer, and the lack of air exchange is causing an accumulation of several air contaminants, perhaps the most important being cigarette smoke.

The present book thus makes a simple but critical examination of the risks of passive smoking, as perceived in the energy-deficient 1980s. The key constituents of tobacco smoke are noted, and the pollutant yield is discussed for various species of such smoke. Observations are related to epidemiological information on the levels of key pollutants observed in public places. Carbon monoxide accumulation is discussed in relation to possible disturbances of psychomotor function and exacerbation of cardiac disease. The acute effects of smoke upon the respiratory tract and on other body systems are considered, and long-term disturbances of health are reviewed in relation to both the general population and sensitive target groups (young children, asthmatics and the elderly). Problems encountered by the fetus and the infant born to a smoking mother are also explored. Final chapters discuss the current attitudes of smokers and non-smokers to the issue of passive smoking, along with possible remedies that will afford a greater measure of protection to the non-smoker.

As in a number of my previous books, personal items of research that are described have been a team effort, conducted in close co-operation with several colleagues and graduate students, both in the Department of Preventive Medicine and Biostatistics and in the Gage Research Institute at the University of Toronto. To ensure a counter-weight to my obvious personal bias, some of those enlisted have themselves been inveterate smokers! Without drawing any embarrassing distinction between representatives of the two factions, I gratefully acknowledge the co-operation of Drs Frances Silverman, P.K. Basu, Andris Rode, Robert LaBarre and Geoffrey Wright, along with Elenor Ponsford, Peter Pimm, Rick Collins, Bruce Erch, S. Jewczyk, J. Onrot and P. Tomlinson. The investigations have profited greatly from the enthusiastic support of Mr Ray Kozan and the York–Toronto Lung Association. There has also been a happy bilingual co-operation with the Departments of Health Sciences and Mathematics in the University of Québec at Trois Rivières, where much of the data processing has been completed.

Many life-long smokers now say (with varying degrees of conviction) that they wish to escape from their addiction. Possibly, a clearer definition of the risks of passive smoking may help them in the realization of this ambition. Social reinforcement is an important reason why many people continue to smoke. If public display of the habit becomes socially-inappropriate behaviour, the ranks of the smokers will quickly diminish. For too long, society has regarded smoking as a harmless foible, or even a foil of graceful living. It is time for it to be exposed as a social menace, endangering the health not only of the addict, but also of his family, friends and acquaintances. Viewed in such terms, cigarettes have no more place in a public restaurant than a spittoon or an open latrine.

I am by nature an optimist. Nevertheless there are limits to my optimism, and I do not believe this book will instantaneously assure smoke-free air in all public buildings. Ideas in public health seem to have an incubation period of at least ten years.

A few years ago, health education was being severely criticized on the basis that repeated preaching of exercise, abstinence from cigarettes and choice of a low-fat diet was having no impact upon public behaviour. Now, exercise facilities are crowded, the proportion of cigarette smokers in all age groups is showing a steady decline, and there is a parallel trend to a decrease of cardiac deaths in 'Western' nations. I am optimistic enough to detect also a trend towards the establishment of smoke-free zones in shops, offices, aircraft, trains and buses. Furthermore, the trend is gathering momentum. If the present book helps forward this important process of social history, my efforts will be well-rewarded.

1 CONSTITUENTS OF TOBACCO SMOKE

The Combustion Process

The nature of the combustion process, and thus the composition of tobacco smoke, varies with the form of tobacco usage (pipe, cigar or cigarette). However, the greatest amount of research to date has been focused upon the machine rolled cigarette.

The four functional components of a modern cigarette are the combustion zone, the pyrolysis zone, the distillation zone and the filter (Hobbs, 1957; Keith, 1972).

Combustion Zone

The combustion zone is the red, glowing tip of the cigarette. Here, burning is relatively complete, the tobacco being converted to simple products such as carbon monoxide, carbon dioxide and water, with extraction of most of the oxygen. During a 'puff', burning occurs mainly at the periphery of the cigarette, close to the paper, while between draws combustion is most marked in the central zone (Egerton *et al.*, 1936). The temperature is highest in the central zone, and it is here that the yield of polycyclic hydrocarbons is greatest (Wynder & Hoffmann, 1967).

Cigarettes vary somewhat in their temperatures of combustion. A high temperature (induced by reflection or insulating ash) causes the cigarette to burn faster, allowing fewer 'puffs' per cigarette. Although the tar formation is increased, the smoker has less time to inhale the toxic material; however, he may feel cheated by the rapidity with which the cigarette disappears. The cone temperatures can be reduced by the use of additives such as sulphur, magnesium carbonate or vanadium pentoxide (Miller *et al.*, 1968). These substances reduce the yield of polycyclic hydrocarbons, but have the practical disadvantage that unless the addict puffs frantically the resultant cigarette extinguishes itself.

Pyrolysis Zone

The pyrolysis zone lies immediately behind the glowing tip of the cigarette. Here a combination of high temperature (600-1050°C, Baker, 1974) and a reducing gas rich in hydrogen encourage both conversion of CO_2 to carbon monoxide (Dudley, 1888) and pyrolysis of the tobacco to a variety of noxious hydrocarbons (Hobbs, 1957; Newsome & Keith, 1965). The hydrocarbons condense on very small nuclei emitted by the combustion zone, yielding an extremely dense smoke cloud (10^8 to 10^{10} per ml) of spherical particles with a relatively uniform size (range 0.2–1.0 μ, median 0.15–0.20 μ on a number average, 0.5–0.6 μ on a mass average; Keith & Derrick, 1960; Kiefer, 1972; Carter & Hasegawa, 1975).

Attempts to check pyrolysis of the tobacco have not been particularly successful. Cigarettes have been designed that fuse to a molten mass, trapping unwanted chemicals, but it is then difficult to draw air through the tube. More complete combustion of the tobacco to carbon dioxide can be encouraged by use of rapidly burning, porous paper (Schur & Rickard, 1960), but the fire extinguishing properties of CO_2 do not commend such modifications to the serious smoker. Newsome & Keith (1965) suggested that with the typical cigarette paper of the era, 30% of the inhaled gas passed through the combustion cone, 15% entered around the cone and 55% of air entered through the wrapper. Smoke dilution has subsequently been encouraged by deliberate perforation of the wrapper. Carried to its logical conclusion, such an arrangement could allow the smoker to breathe almost pure air, while liberally polluting the room in which he or she is seated. Dilution has more effect upon the gaseous constituents of the smoke than upon the nicotine and particulate count.

Distillation Zone

The temperature of the smoke drops quite rapidly to about 40°C as it passes through the cigarette (Touey & Mumpower, 1957; Neurath *et al.*, 1966). Cooling favours the condensation of smoke constituents with a high boiling point; there is also a tendency for coagulation of the smoke particles (Kiefer, 1972). Nevertheless, little mechanical filtration occurs, and in the region immediately adjacent to the pyrolysis zone the temperature remains high enough for 20–30% of nicotine, additives such as menthol and other compounds such as dotriacontane (Carpenter *et al.*, 1970; Wakeham, 1972), to distil into the smoke without alteration of chemical composition. In this segment, smoke can also diffuse through the wrapper into the room, while the material inhaled by the smoker can be diluted by room air (Schur & Rickard, 1960; Owen & Reynolds, 1967). It is further possible to change the characteristics of the smoke in this zone by pre-treatment of the tobacco, or replacement of some of the tobacco by a less toxic 'filler'.

Figure 1.1: Smoke Removal (% of Weighable Material) Seen with Filters of 20 mm and 30 mm Length in Relation to Pressure Drop during Standard 'Puff'

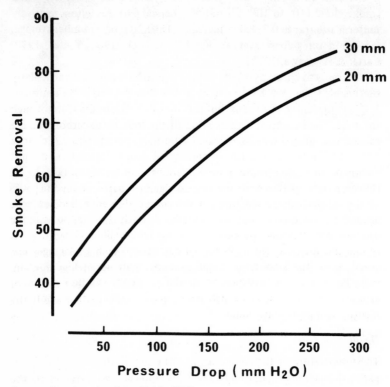

Source: Based on data from Keith, 1972.

Filter

The great majority of modern cigarettes finally incorporate a 'filter'. The purpose of this is to trap selective particulate matter and toxic components of the gas phase. The efficiency of various designs of filter ranges from 20 to 75%, depending upon the 'puff' resistance the smoker is prepared to accept (Figure 1.1). The pressure drop can be diminished by incorporating an air vent into the filter; such vents not only dilute the smoke, but also slow its passage through the filter, encouraging particle deposition. Depending on the routing of the air stream, previously deposited volatile constituents may also be re-incorporated into the smoke. The filtration of smoke particles,

Table 1.1: Efficiency of Filters in Removing Smoke, Nicotine and Tar

Constituent	Constant A	Constant B	Constant C
Smoke	-1.54×10^{-2}	-0.96×10^{-8}	-2.10×10^{-2}
Nicotine	-0.38×10^{-2}	-1.05×10^{-8}	-1.82×10^{-2}
Tar	-1.00×10^{-2}	-0.85×10^{-8}	-2.59×10^{-2}

The equation for removal efficiency (E) is:

$$\log_e \left(1 - \frac{E}{100}\right) = (A \cdot L) + (B \cdot \Delta P \cdot C^4) + (D \cdot L / \delta)$$

where L is the filter length in mm, ΔP is the filter pressure drop (mm H_2O at 17.5 ml sec^{-1} flow), C is the filter circumference and δ is the fibre denier for filament, in g.

Source: Based on data from Keith, 1972.

nicotine and tar normally proceeds roughly in parallel (Table 1.1). However, it is possible to influence the relative absorption of vapours having an intermediate volatility. Unfortunately, such compounds give flavour to the smoke, and for this reason an effective filter may be unacceptable to the dedicated smoker. Nevertheless, selectivity is technically possible. By use of a carbon filter, for example, one can achieve a tenfold selectivity in the removal of irritants such as acrolein. Cellulose acetate filters, in contrast, give a selective extraction of phenol (twofold to threefold) and other polar compounds, while filters containing hydrocarbon polymers are particularly effective in removing non-polar compounds.

Conclusion

The foregoing discussion indicates a wide possible variation in the composition of tobacco smoke. Furthermore, the average composition has undergone a progressive secular change in response to the pressure of governmental legislation, and increasingly desperate attempts by the manufacturers of cigarettes to convince smokers that their addiction is a harmless pleasure.

Techniques of Smoke Production and Collection

It is usual to generate the smoke for laboratory experiments using some type of smoking machine. This implies a need to determine the smoking pattern of the average consumer, followed by reproduction of this pattern using a suitable mechanical device.

Table 1.2: Characteristics Selected for the Machine-smoking of
Cigarettes

| Variable | Machine characteristics | | Smoking behaviour |
	Median	Range	Range
'Puff' volume (ml)	35	25–40	17–73
'Puff' frequency (min⁻¹)	1	1–4	0.8–2.6
'Puff' duration (sec)	2	1–3	0.9–3.2
Butt length (mm)	23[a]	15–30	—

Note: a. 30 mm adopted in North American machines.
Source: Based on data collected by Wynder & Hoffmann, 1967; Wakeham, 1972.

Smoking Pattern

Attempts to determine the normal pattern of cigarette smoking have
included surreptitious observation of smokers in bars and restaurants,
and deliberate videotaping of smokers seated in front of a television
camera. Neither approach has successfully explored the full range of
situations in which cigarettes are consumed.

Variables examined have included 'puff' volume, 'puff' frequency,
'puff' duration and butt length (Table 1.2). Schur & Rickards (1957)
directed occasional 'puffs' into a kymograph, deducing a 'puff' volume
of 37 ± 10 ml. Mitchell (1962) had his subjects inhale air through a
small pneumotachometer and, perhaps for this reason, recorded a larger
volume of 45 ± 10 ml. Keith (1972) incorporated a hot wire anemometer
into a cigarette holder, and from this device estimated the 'puff' volume
at 44 ml. Other figures have been based upon the number of 'puffs'
obtained from a cigarette (25 ml, Bentley & Burgan, 1961) or the
amount of tobacco consumed (35 ml, Waltz & Hauserman, 1960). With
a few exceptions, most investigators currently accept 35 ml as the
standard 'puff'. However, it is likely that average volumes have increased
as cigarettes have become milder. Recent observations suggest that a
'puff' volume of 45–50 ml is realistic for the current generation of
smokers (Rickert *et al.*, in preparation).

The 'puff' duration observed in early studies was 1.6–1.9 seconds
(Schur & Rickards, 1957; Mitchell, 1962; Keith, 1972), similar to the
2.0 seconds adopted in most smoking machines. Again, Rickert *et al.*
(in preparation) suggest that with the introduction of milder cigarettes,
the 'puff' duration has now increased to an average of 2.4 seconds.

The 'puff' frequency of most smoking machines is an arbitrary one
per minute, although both early (Bentley & Burgan, 1961; Keith, 1972)
and more recent observations of smokers (Rickert *et al.*, in preparation)

have set the actual inter-puff interval at an average of about 45 seconds.

The butt length varies widely with socio-economic circumstances from a low of 15 mm to a high of 31 mm (Wynder & Hoffmann, 1967). The current generation of North American smoking machines generally assumes a 30 mm figure, but the populations on which this is based have included employees of cigarette manufacturing companies who received an allowance of 'free' or low cost cigarettes. A recent study of 10,000 butts in Canada (Rickert *et al.*, in preparation) indicated a substantially shorter butt length (average 23 mm).

Smoking Machines

The basic elements of a smoking machine are: (i) a constant speed pump or a vacuum system; (ii) a series of cigarette holders; and (iii) an arrangement of solenoid-operated valves that time 'puff'-duration. Condensers may be arranged beyond the cigarette holders to trap smoke drawn through the cigarettes and, for some applications, the apparatus may be enclosed in order to collect 'side-stream' smoke.

One drawback to all such devices is a complicated arrangement of plumbing; this may in itself modify smoke composition. Devices with rigid stainless steel pipes also generate a 'puff' with a 'square' slow profile, in contrast to the triangular profile anticipated in a typical smoker. Furthermore, unless suction can be increased, the 'puff' volume will diminish as the cigarette becomes clogged and the draw resistance rises. Finally, the 'standard' pattern of smoking provided by the usual machine is inappropriate for the evaluation of cigars and cigarillos (International Committee, 1974).

Smoke Constituents

General Considerations

It is usual to distinguish the discontinuous or particulate phase of cigarette smoke from the continuous or gaseous phase (the latter including all components that are volatile at $30°C$; Wynder & Hoffmann, 1967). Nevertheless, a number of the important constituents of cigarette smoke are found in both phases of the smoke (US Surgeon General, 1972, 1979). Several review articles (Johnstone & Plimmer, 1959; Stedman, 1968; Neurath, 1972; Falk, 1977) have already listed over 2,000 potentially toxic compounds; moreover, gas chromatograph tracing suggests that other materials yet remain to be identified (Wakeham, 1972).

Table 1.3: Principal Constituents of Cigarette Smoke

Constituent	Mass (mg per cigarette)	Mass in effluent (per cent)	Gas phase composition volume per cent
Particulate matter (including condensed water)	40.6	8.2	—
Nitrogen	295.4	59.0	67.2
Oxygen	66.8	13.4	13.3
Carbon dioxide	68.1	13.6	9.8
Carbon monoxide	16.2	3.2	3.7
Hydrogen	0.7	0.1	2.2
Argon	5.0	1.0	0.8
Methane	1.3	0.3	0.5
Water vapour	5.8	1.2	—
Hydrocarbons	2.5	0.5	—
Carbonyls	1.9	0.4	—
Hydrogen cyanide	0.3	0.1	—
Other gases	1.0	0.2	—

(handwritten: pie chart)

Source: After Keith & Tesh, 1965. Observations based on 10 puffs, each of 38.9 ml volume (85 mm cigarette smoked to 30 mm butt length).

(handwritten: act-amounts may have changed, although constituents same p2a)

Table 1.4: Influence of Smoking Pattern on the Composition of Cigarette Smoke

Type of cigarette	Standard smoking machine			Modified smoking pattern		
	Tar (mg)	CO (mg)	Nicotine (mg)	Tar (mg)	CO (mg)	Nicotine (mg)
Players Regular Filter	17	17	1.2	35	30	2.4
Viscount Extra-Light King-Size Filter	1	1	0.07	12	23	0.6

Source: Based on data from Rickert, 1981, per cigarette.

The principal constituents include particulate matter, various gases, hydrocarbons, carbonyls and hydrogen cyanide (Table 1.3). In terms of health, the US Surgeon General (1972) has distinguished:

(i) the most likely hazards (Table 1.4 — carbon monoxide, nicotine and 'tar' — the particulate residue remaining after elimination of nicotine and water);

Table 1.5: Probable Contributors to the Health Hazards of Cigarette Smoke

Compound	Likely yield per cigarette (mg)	(ppm)	Threshold limit[a] (ppm)	(mg'm^{-3})
Acrolein	0.045–0.140	52– 160	0.1	0.25
Phenol	0.009–0.202	6– 135[b]	5	19
Cresol[c]	0.068–0.097	39– 56[b]	5	22
Hydrogen cyanide	0.100–0.400	237– 948	10	11
Nitric oxide	0 –0.600	0–1280	25	30
Nitrogen dioxide	0 –0.010	0– 14	5	9

Notes: a. For 8-hour work day.
    b. By mass.
    c. Distributed in roughly equal proportions between o-, m- and p- isomers.
Source: Based partly on US Surgeon General, 1972.

(ii) probable health hazards (Table 1.5 – acrolein, cresol, hydrogen cyanide, nitric oxide, nitrogen dioxide and phenol);
(iii) possible health hazards (Table 1.6 – acetaldehyde, acetone, acetonitrile, acrylonitrile, ammonia, benzene, 2,3 butadione, butylamine, carbon dioxide, crotononitrile, dimethylamine, DDT, endrin, ethylamine, formaldehyde, furfural, hydrogen sulphide, hydroquinone, methacrolein, methyl alcohol, methylamine, nickel compounds and pyridine).

Traces of other toxic material have also been described, including various heavy metals, insecticides, fungicides, fungal products and viruses.

Carbon Monoxide

The yield of carbon monoxide ranges from 5.2–21.4 mg per cigarette, the gas phase concentration ranging from 2.7 to 6.0% (Wynder & Hoffmann, 1967; US Surgeon General, 1972). The CO concentration of inhaled smoke approximately doubles from the first few 'puffs' (2.4–3.1%) to the final 'puffs' (5.0–5.3%), because less air can enter through the paper of a shorter cigarette (Mumpower *et al.*, 1962; Newsome & Keith, 1965). Similar variations of CO concentrations occur if the porosity of the cigarette paper is modified.

The moisture content and weight of the cigarette have little effect on CO concentrations in the smoke (Mumpower *et al.*, 1962). Data are also comparable for filter and non-filter cigarettes, but CO

Table 1.6: Possible Contributors to the Health Hazards of Cigarette Smoke

Compound	Likely yield per cigarette (mg)	(ppm)	Threshold limit (ppm)	(mg'm⁻³)
Acetaldehyde	0.18 – 1.44	262-2095	200	360
Acetone	0.088– 0.65	97-717	1000	2400
Acetonitrile	0.14 – 0.20	219-312	40	70
Acrylonitrile	0.010– 0.015	9-18	20	45
Ammonia	0.06 – 0.33	226-621	50	35
Benzene	0.012– 0.10	10-41	25	80
2,3 Butanedione	0.043– 0.20	25-119	–	–
Butylamine	0.003	1.5	5	15
Carbon dioxide	23.1 –78.3	33,600-113,890	5000	9000
Crotononitrile	0.004	3.8	–	–
Dimethylamine	0.010– 0.011	10-11	10	18
DDT	0– 0.77×10^{-3}	–	–	1
Endrin	0.06×10^{-3}	0.01	–	0.1
Ethylamine	0.010– 0.011	14-15	10	18
Formaldehyde	0.020– 0.041	22-43	5	6
Furfural	0.045– 0.110	30-73	5	20
Hydrogen sulphide	0.012– 0.035	23-66	10	15
Hydroquinone	0.083	48	–	2
Methacrolein	0.009– 0.011	–	–	–
Methyl alcohol	0.09– 0.30	180-600	200	260
Methylamine	0.020– 0.022	40-44	10	12
Nickel compounds	0– 0.58×10^{-3}	–	–	1
Pyridine	0.025– 0.218	22-177	5	15

Source: Based partly on US Surgeon General, 1972.

concentrations are higher in the early 'puffs' from regular as opposed to King-Sized cigarettes (Robinson & Forbes, 1975). Furthermore, the percentage of CO inhaled increases greatly with 'puff' volume; for instance, at the eighth puff, concentrations are 1.3% for 20 ml, 4.4% for 35 ml and 5.3% for 60 ml 'puff' volume (Mumpower *et al.*, 1962).

Nicotine

The nicotine yield depends in part upon the type of tobacco that is used in manufacture of the cigarette. The nicotine content of the leaf is increased by a boron deficiency in the soil (Steinberg & Jeffrey, 1956), but can be reduced by genetic manipulation of the tobacco plant and subsequent flue-curing (Weybrew *et al.*, 1972). US Burley tobacco often contains 9–10% nicotine, but in Turkish tobacco, the nicotine content may be as low as 0.5–1.0% (Wynder & Hoffmann, 1967). Other variables influencing the composition of the smoke include: (i) the proportion of nicotine that is pyrolysed to pyridine, myosmine, bipyridyl, heterocyclic compounds such as dibenzacridines and dibenzocarbazole, and aromatic hydrocarbons (Jarboe & Rosene, 1961; Wynder & Hoffmann, 1967; US Surgeon General, 1972); (ii) the extent of nicotine absorption in the filter; and (iii) dilution of the smoke by any air vents in the paper or the filter.

Manufacturers have progressively reduced the nicotine yield of cigarettes over the last 20 years. Changes have been particularly marked since it became mandatory to publish information. Some cigarettes are still noted as delivering 2.5 mg of nicotine, but typical figures for 'medium' and 'light' cigarettes now range from 1.2 mg (Players Regular Filter) to 0.07 mg (Viscount Extra-Light King-Size Filter). Such statistics are based upon combustion in a standard smoking machine. It is probable that consumers have modified their smoking habits as the nicotine yield has fallen. Given a likely current smoking pattern (a 2.4 second 'puff', a 47.5 ml volume and a 44 second inter-puff interval), the nicotine delivered to the smoker would be doubled for normal cigarettes and would increase almost tenfold for ventilated cigarettes (Table 1.4).

Particulate Matter

Wet particulate matter may be defined as that fraction of smoke separated from the gas phase by use of a specific Cambridge filter (CM-113). It comprises 0.2–9.0% by weight of 'mainstream' smoke and includes not only 'tar' but also nicotine, moisture and various absorbed vapours. The 'tar' can be separated from the gaseous components of tobacco smoke, using cold-traps or condensate; it contains a number of polycyclic aromatic hydrocarbons with known carcinogenic activity. Some are present in too low a concentration to assume total responsibility for carcinogenesis, although they could play a role as tumour initiators or co-carcinogens. For other compounds, such as beta-naphthylamine, there is no known safe level of exposure, so that the traces encountered by the smoker and his friends must be viewed with grave suspicion (Tables 1.7 and 1.8).

The amount of tar delivered by a given tobacco depends upon the variety of plant, the stalk position of the leaf that has been processed and the grade of the blend (Tso & Gori, 1972). A coarse-cut blend smoulders more between 'puffs', producing a larger amount of tar. Some tar condenses in the butt, but can be redistilled; this factor, along with diminishing air dilution, causes a progressive increase of tar delivery

Table 1.7: Polycyclic Aromatic Hydrocarbons with Tumour Initiating or Co-carcinogenic Activity

Compound	Concentrations in cigarette smoke (μg per cigarette)	Relative activity as carcinogen
Tumour initiators		
Benzo (a) pyrene	10– 50	3+
5 methylchrysene	0.6	3+
Dibenz (a,h) anthracene	40	2+
Benzo (b) fluoranthrene	30	2+
Benzo (j) fluoranthrene	60	2+
Dibenzo (a,h) pyrene	?	2+
Dibenzo (a,j) pyrene	?	2+
Indeno (1,2,3-cd) pyrene	4	+
Benzo (c) phenanthrene	?	+
Benzo (a) anthracene	40– 70	+
Chrysene	40– 60	?
Benzo (e) pyrene	5– 40	?
2,3-methylchrysene	7	+
1,6-methylchrysene	10	–
2-methylfluoranthrene	30	+
3-methylfluoranthrene	40	?
Dibenz (a,c) anthracene	?	?
Co-carcinogens		
Pyrene	50–200	–
Methylpyrene	50–300	–
Fluoranthrene	100–260	–
Benzo (g,h,i) perylene	60	–

Source: Based on data from Hoffmann *et al.*, 1976.

Table 1.8: Relative Yield of Toxic Hydrocarbons (μg per 100 g of Tobacco Consumed)

Constituent	Cigarettes	Cigars	Light pipe tobacco
Acenaphthylene	5.0	1.6	29.1
Anthracene	10.9	11.9	110.0
Pyrene	12.5	17.6	75.5
3-4 benzpyrene	0.9	3.4	8.5

Source: Based on data from Campbell & Lindsey, 1957.

with successive 'puffs' (Wynder & Hoffmann, 1967). The yield of tar is diminished if the temperature in the pyrolysis zone can be reduced; certain additives (nickel and cobalt powder) also diminish the formation of benz (α) pyrene (Bentley & Burgan, 1960).

There has been substantial governmental pressure to market low tar cigarettes in recent years. Current figures for 'medium' and 'light' cigarettes range from 1 to 20 mg when a cigarette is burnt in a conventional smoking machine, and from 12 to 35 mg when the machine is modified to represent modern smoking patterns. In Canada, the sales-weighted nominal tar delivery has dropped about 30% over the past decade. Similarly, the US sales-weighted average decreased from 39 to 17 mg between 1957 and 1976 (Wakeham, 1976). Nevertheless, there remains a substantial segment of the population who try to create a 'macho' image for themselves by smoking 'strong' cigarettes, with a high output of tars.

Acrolein

Acrolein, or acrylic aldehyde (CH_2:CH. CHO) is a pungent gas, toxic to the tracheal ciliae. It is formed by the decomposition of glycerin. Lesser amounts of other unsaturated aldehydes (methacrolein, crotonaldehyde and 1-butenone) are also present in tobacco smoke (Grob, 1962). The acrolein delivery varies with leaf characteristics such as nitrate, wax, polyphenol and alkaloid content (Tso & Gori, 1972). Acrolein can be selectively removed from inhaled smoke using carbon filters, but unfortunately this does little to check contamination of room air (Williamson *et al.*, 1965). As with most of the other toxic compounds, the concentration of acrolein in the inhaled smoke rises with a decrease of cigarette length; typical figures for total yield are 45 to 140 μg per cigarette.

Phenols

Phenol (C_6H_5 OH), the three isomers of cresol ($CH_3C_6H_4$ OH) and other phenols such as catechol, hydroquinone and resorcinol are all constituents of cigarette smoke that reach concentrations of concern for health (Herrmann, 1964). The phenols are toxic to ciliae, and directly or indirectly can contribute to carcinogenic change in exposed cells. The primary sources include glucose, sucrose, starch, cellulose, pectin, the polyphenol rutin and the hydrocarbons docosane and tetracosane; pyrolysis converts small amounts of each of these compounds to phenols (Spears *et al.*, 1965; Schlotzhauer *et al.*, 1972; Wakeham, 1972). The yield of phenol itself is greatest with Oriental tobacco (0.24 to 0.36 mg per cigarette) and least with Burley tobacco (0.04 mg per cigarette). The delivery of cresol (all isomers) ranges from 0.07 to 0.1 mg per cigarette (US Surgeon General, 1972). Up to 50% of phenols are removed by cellulose acetate filters (Williamson *et al.*, 1965).

Hydrocyanic Acid

The presence of hydrogen cyanide (HCN) in tobacco smoke (Elmenhorst & Schultz, 1968) was first acknowledged as early as 1858; it is formed from amino acids and protein (Johnson *et al.*, 1973a). Excretion of hydrogen thiocyanate in the saliva provides one simple method of estimating smoke exposure, since the half-life of the thiocyanate that is formed during detoxification of HCN is some 14 days (Vogt *et al.*, 1977). There is about a threefold increase of HCN concentration in the inhaled smoke from the first to the last 'puff'; in addition to the usual decrease in air dilution, there is some evidence that filters become saturated with HCN before the cigarette is extinguished (Williamson & Allman, 1964). Nevertheless, the amount delivered to the smoker (0.1 to 0.4 mg per cigarette) can be reduced appreciably by use of charcoal filters. In cigar smoke, 10 to 30% of the gas reported as HCN may actually be cyanogen (Brunnemann *et al.*, 1977c).

Oxides of Nitrogen

Tobacco smoke contains various oxides of nitrogen (NO_x-nitric oxide and nitrogen dioxide, along with small amounts of nitrous oxide and methyl nitrite; Haagen-Smit *et al.*, 1959; Norman & Keith, 1965). The main constituent of fresh smoke is nitric oxide (NO, half-life about 10 minutes); as this gas ages, nitrogen dioxide (NO_2) is formed. Both NO and NO_2 are toxic in their own right, but they also facilitate the formation of carcinogenic nitrosamines. The primary source of the oxides of nitrogen is nitrate. The leaf content ranges from 0 to 6% in different varieties of tobacco, depending upon the nature of the soil and the amount of chemical fertilizer that has been used. Occasionally, nitrates have been deliberately added to cigarettes of dubious quality in order to encourage them to burn. Fast-burning cigarettes deliver 3 times more NO_x than slowly burning varieties. Within a given tobacco plant, the nitrate content is least in the tips of the leaves (Neurath & Ehmke, 1964). The nitric oxide content of the smoke varies from 0 to 0.6 mg per cigarette, and depending upon the extent of aging of the smoke, the NO_2 production is 0 to 0.01 mg per cigarette.

Other Constituents

Other possible harmful constituents (Table 1.6) may be grouped into compounds containing nitrogen (amines, nitriles, alkaloids and hetero-cyclics), compounds containing oxygen (alcohols, phenols, carbonyl compounds, acids, heterocyclics and carbon dioxide), compounds containing sulphur, hydrocarbons (alkanes, alkenes, alkines, simple and polycyclic aromatics), trace elements, pesticides, fungi and viruses.

Compounds Containing Nitrogen

Ammonia (Neurath *et al.*, 1966a; Johnson *et al.*, 1973b), primary amines (methylamine, ethylamine and butylamine) and secondary amines (dimethylamine and pyrrolidine) have all been detected in cigarette smoke in relatively small amounts (Neurath, 1969). The secondary amines are of particular concern, not only in their own right, but also as potential precursors of the highly carcinogenic nitrosamines (Magee & Barnes, 1966; Fine *et al.*, 1975; Brunnemann *et al.*, 1977b):

$$2 \frac{R_1}{R_2} > N - H + NO + NO_2 \rightleftarrows \quad 2 \frac{R_1}{R_2} > N - NO + H_2O \quad \text{and}$$

$$\frac{R_1}{R_2} > N - H + H_3CO - NO \rightleftarrows \quad \frac{R_1}{R_2} > N - NO + CH_3OH$$

The use of sucker-inhibiting agents such as maleic hydrazide and enzymatic curing also encourage nitrosamine formation (Hecht *et al.*, 1975; Schmeltz & Hoffmann, 1977; Schmeltz *et al.*, 1977). Concentrations of these hazardous compounds are thus up to ten times higher in cigar tobacco than in cigarette tobacco.

Traces of aromatic amines (aniline and naphthylamine) have been detected in cigarette smoke, but concentrations seem insufficient to contribute to carcinogenesis (Neurath *et al.*, 1966a; Masuda & Hoffmann, 1969). The related mutagenic amino β carbolines (Sugimara *et al.*, 1976) may be much more dangerous. Hydrogen cyanide has been discussed above. Other nitriles found in cigarette smoke include acetonitrile, proprionitrile and irritant unsaturated nitriles such as acrylonitrile, crotononitrile and methacrylonitrile (Grob, 1962; Schmeltz & Hoffmann, 1977). This last group of compounds is formed during the pyrolysis of pyridine and related compounds and concentrations of most items substantially exceed the industrial threshold limit. The principal alkaloid of tobacco smoke is nicotine, but small amounts of nornicotine, anabasine, anatabine and myosmine are also found. Cotinine (57 μg cigarette) is formed by oxidation of nicotine, and it has been suggested that this last compound is carcinogenic (Truhaut *et al.*, 1964). Pyridine is an aromatic base found in the particulate phase of tobacco smoke. It is the main product of nicotine pyrolysis (Neurath, 1969). Many heterocyclic compounds are produced in smaller amounts, including quinoline, indole, pyrrol, skatole, pyrazine, dibenzacridine and dibenzcarbazole. The last two compounds listed are known to have carcinogenic properties, while certain of the quinolines can also induce mutations.

Compounds Containing Oxygen

The vapour phase of tobacco smoke contains fair amounts of methanol (Grob, 1962; Stedman, 1968). Long-chained primary alcohols are found in the particulate phase. Menthol is sometimes added for flavouring; the compound seems to be vapourized without chemical change. Sterols (stigmasterol, β sitosterol, compesterol and cholesterol) are also transferred unchanged to the smoke (Grunwald *et al.*, 1971). Simple phenols have been discussed above. The polyphenol scopoletin is found in the smoke if the tobacco plants have been grown on boron deficient soil (Watanabe *et al.*, 1961); another prominent polyphenol (catechol) could serve as a tumour promoter and carcinogen (Carter & Hasegawa, 1975). The carbonyl compounds (acetaldehyde, formaldehyde, furfural, acetone, methacrolein, 2-3 butanedione) contribute not only to the irritant, cilio-toxic properties of tobacco smoke, but also to its taste (Stedman, 1968). They are formed from carbohydrates by a combination of pyrolysis and steam distillation. There is about a 50% increase in the inhaled concentrations of acetone and acetaldehyde from 'puff' two to 'puff' twelve. Some of the formaldehyde is carried on particulate matter, and is thus removed by a cellulose acetate filter. Deactivated carbon filters provide an effective method of removing carbonyl compounds from the gas phase of the smoke. The carbonyl yield is greater from Bright than from Burley tobacco, due to the high content of reducing sugars in the former variety. Dry cigarettes also generate more aldehydes. Unsaturated aldehydes such as acrolein have been discussed above. Volatile fatty acids (acetic, formic and beta methyl valeric) and non volatile fatty acids (stearic, palmitic, myristic, lauric, linoleic, linolenic) find their way into the smoke, but do not seem a specific health hazard. Heterocyclic compounds include furan, 2-methylfuran and 2-5 dimethylfuran (Grob, 1962). Their biological significance is uncertain; concentrations depend on the sugar content of the tobacco (Falk, 1977). Carbon dioxide, although a major constituent of tobacco smoke, is unlikely to present a serious hazard to a healthy person. It is included in Table 1.6 merely because it could add to respiratory problems in a patient with chronic chest disease.

Compounds Containing Sulphur

Hydrogen sulphide, although only present in low concentration, exceeds industrially permitted limits. Other sulphur compounds that have been described in tobacco smoke include carbonyl sulphide, methyl thionitrile, carbon disulphide, thiophene and sulphur dioxide (Grob, 1962; Elmenhorst & Schultz, 1968; Guerin, 1971; Horton & Guerin, 1974).

Hydrocarbons

Volatile hydrocarbons are derived from the waxy coating of the leaves (Stedman, 1968). Components found in tobacco smoke include alkanes such as methane and ethane, alkenes such as ethylene and propene, dienes such as 2 methylbutadiene (isoprene), alkines such as acetylene, cyclic hydrocarbons such as cyclohexane and aromatic hydrocarbons such as benzene, toluene and xylene (Sugimura *et al.*, 1976). Benzene is the one compound in this group where the possibility of toxicity has been raised (Grob, 1962; Elmenhorst & Schultz, 1968); workers exposed to benzene have an increased risk of leukaemia. The polycyclic aromatics are of particular concern as carcinogens: compounds of this class that have been noted in smoke include derivatives of indane, indene and fluorene, methylfluoranthrenes, benz-pyrenes, benz-fluoranthrenes, indenopyrene, methylchrysenes and benzanthracenes (Ayres & Thornton, 1965; Wynder & Hoffmann, 1967). The yield of such dangerous constituents depends primarily upon the cellulose, lignin and pectin content of the tobacco leaf (Gilbert & Lindsey, 1957; Wakeham, 1972), with contributions from leaf lipids (Schlotzhauer *et al.*, 1972) such as oils, waxes and resins. Various terpenoids give flavour to tobacco smoke, and some cyclic isoprenoids may be active as tumour promoters (Stedman, 1968).

Trace Elements

Certain of the trace elements commonly found in tobacco (iron, antimony, zinc and selenium) are only transferred in small amounts to the smoke. Mercury (1-3 ppm in the smoke from some Japanese cigarettes) is derived from the paper used in wrapper manufacture (Andrew & Harriss, 1971). Other trace elements that are of concern include lead (from lead arsenate sprays; Daff & Kennaway, 1950), nickel carbonyl (from nickel additives; Szadkowski *et al.*, 1969),

[210]polonium (derived from the soil and air; Ferri & Baratta, 1966), [226]radium (from phosphorus fertilizers; Tso, 1977), [210]lead and cadmium (Szadkowski *et al.*, 1969).

Pesticides

Various pesticides such as arsenic, endrin and DDT have appeared in cigarette smoke at different points in history. The use of arsenate sprays was discouraged from about 1950, and the discovery of dangerous levels of endrin in tobacco smoke prompted the elimination of endrin as a pesticide in the US from 1964. DDD and DDT are also no longer used on tobacco crops. Substantial losses of the newer insecticides occur during flue-curing of the tobacco, and pyrolysis causes decomposition of much of the residue (for example, carbaryl, 99%; endosulphan, 99%; Guthion, 99%; Felodrin, 95%; Malathion, 92%; Guthrie, 1968, 1973; Henry & Thirion, 1970). However, herbicides such as metobromuron (broken down to 4-bromoaniline) remain a potential problem (Corbaz *et al.*, 1969).

Fungi and Viruses

Tobacco leaf is often contaminated by fungal products, including carcinogenic aflatoxins (Forgacs & Carll, 1966; Pattee, 1969) and by the tobacco mosaic virus (Chyle *et al.*, 1971); however, the virus is partially destroyed by the fermentation processes used in the production of cigar and pipe tobacco, and many authors believe that the aflatoxins are also decomposed as the tobacco is burnt.

Conclusion

The smoker is exposed to an alarming variety of noxious chemical and biological materials. Further, the concentrations of the inhaled compounds often substantially exceeds the limits permitted for industrial exposures to the same substances.

Such personal air pollution does not seem the most intelligent form of behaviour. At the same time, it would be rash to conclude that all of the materials identified in tobacco smoke present a hazard to health. Even the most hardened smoker inhales only about 500 ml of smoke from each cigarette, or some 20 litres per day (given a consumption of 40 cigarettes). The threshold dose needed for a biological response is thus that associated with a 3- to 4-minute rather than an 8-hour exposure.

As we shall see in the next chapter, the doses to which the passive smoker is exposed are even lower, and only a few of the 2,000 potentially hazardous chemicals are an actual threat to health.

2 POLLUTANT YIELD OF TOBACCO

In this chapter, we will look briefly at the pollutant yield from different types of tobacco (cigarette, cigar and pipe) and we will examine differences between sidestream and mainstream smoke.

Types of Tobacco

General Considerations

The chemical characteristics of tobacco depend upon the variety of tobacco plant, the environment in which it is grown, the part of the plant that is cut and the method of curing (Wynder & Hoffmann, 1967; Tso & Gori, 1972). There is potential for a threefold variation in sterols, a fivefold variation in phenols, a tenfold variation in nitrates and a thirtyfold variation in alkaloid content.

Commercial tobacco plants are all variants of the species *Nicotiana tabacum*. This has been modified to resist local diseases, and sometimes to reduce the nicotine or tar generating properties of the leaf.

Environmental factors influencing the chemical composition of the leaf include the soil texture, the availability of minerals, organic matter and water, plus appropriate conditions of light and temperature (Tso, 1975). If the soil provides little nitrogen, acetate from the tricarboxylic acid cycle is used to produce such substances as carbohydrates, fats, oils, resins and polyterpines. Oriental tobaccos, for example, are usually grown on a poor soil in areas of limited rainfall. The amount of nicotine is then low, while the gum content is high. The Oriental product is commonly treated with goat or sheep manure, and this tends to give it a high chlorine content.

Cuttings from the tobacco plant are classified in terms of their position on the stem. Commencing at the base, subdivisions include scrape trash and trash lugs (used for granulated smoking); sand lugs, good lugs and best leaf (used for cigarettes); second leaf (used for chewing and wrappers); tips and green tips (used for chewing and fillers). The carbohydrate content decreases on moving up the plant from the best leaf, but the nicotine and nitrogen content increase. In some regions of the world, the natural processes of growth and maturation are modified by 'pruning' (removal of leaves as they mature), 'topping' (removal of the main shoot) or 'suckering' (removal of axillary shoots). Furthermore, if the leaf is separated from the stem ('pruning'), the leaf contents cannot drain into the stalk during curing. Combustibility decreases with higher leaf position, and this inevitably modifies the characteristics of the smoke that is produced. High combustibility is associated with a lesser yield of total particulates, nicotine, cresols, phenols, hydrogen cyanide and benzanthracene, but a greater output of acetaldehyde, acrolein and carbon monoxide.

The 'curing' of tobacco involves dehydration of the leaf, destruction of chlorophyll and other chemical changes, including the hydrolysis of starch to simple sugars, of proteins to amino acids and of pectins to pectic acid, uronic acid and methanol. Flue-curing requires hanging of the tobacco in a humid barn at a temperature rising from 30 to 75°C over five to seven days. After several months of bulk storage, the tobacco is redried, and it may then be aged for as long as two to three years, causing a further slow change in its chemical characteristics. Burley and cigar tobaccos are air-cured; in this process, whole plants wilt in the field, and are then stored in sheds with a regulated flow of air for 30 to 40 days. Chemical changes include hydrolysis, followed by an oxidation of sugars to acids. There is also an oxidation and polymerization of some phenols and a decrease of alkaloids. After a year or so of storage, cigar tobacco undergoes several cycles of fermentation in rooms held at 45°C and 60% relative humidity. The action of naturally occurring oxidative and hydrolytic enzymes is thus supplemented by the enzymes of bacteria and fungi which multiply in the warm and moist environment. The result is a dramatic decrease in the sugar content of the tobacco, with smaller reductions in the content of organic and amino acids. Other changes include a breakdown of pectins, hemi-celluloses, gums, resins and volatile oils. Oriental tobacco is harvested by 'priming' and the leaves are cured by allowing them to dry in the sun. After tight baling, they are stored for about two years, and a slow fermentation occurs within the bales. The nicotine content of Oriental tobacco is low because close-spacing of the plants and shallow soil limits root growth. Flue-cured tobacco accumulates phenol from the smoke of hardwood fires. It is used mainly for the manufacture of snuff, and is rarely incorporated into cigarettes. In recent years, mechanization has aroused interest in 'homogenized leaf curing'; the various chemical changes discussed above then take place in a homogenized tobacco slurry, and attempts can be made to remove undesirable constituents before the tobacco is reconstituted as a sheet (Tso *et al.*, 1975).

Cigarettes

Traditionally, cigarettes have been manufactured from varying proportions of Virginian (flue-cured), Burley, Maryland and Oriental tobaccos. The characteristics of the smoke from these several varieties reflect underlying differences of chemical composition. Nitrogen compounds impart 'strength', tannins and resins — aromaticity, sugars — mildness and cell membrane constituents — 'sharpness' of odour. The best leaf of Virginian tobacco inparts what the smoker regards as a pleasant flavour and aroma, although if basal and tip-leaves are added, the smoke can become more pungent. Virginian tobacco has a high sugar content, and a medium to low content of nicotine, nitrogenous compounds and acids. Burley tobacco is a major constituent of most cigarettes, since it burns well, produces a mild smoke and absorbs flavouring agents and humectants; again, the strength and pungency of the smoke are increased if the upper leaves are included. Burley tobacco has a low carbohydrate content, but is rich in nicotine, nitrogenous compounds and acids. It also yields more carbon monoxide than Bright tobacco (Osborne *et al.*, 1956). Maryland tobacco burns well, but the smoke is not pleasing to most smokers; both nicotine and carbohydrate content are low, while nitrogenous compounds and acids are present in moderate concentrations. Oriental tobaccos are added to blends mainly for their aroma; the nicotine content of the Oriental product is low, carbohydrate and nitrogenous compounds are present in average concentrations and acid concentrations are relatively high.

In recent years, an ever increasing proportion of reconstituted tobacco sheet has been added to most blends (Moshey, 1967; Mattina & Selke, 1975). Paper-making techniques are commonly used to form a web of tobacco, but less commonly adhesives such as hydrocolloid gum are added to help the formation of a continuous sheet of tobacco. The reconstituted sheet is chopped into leaflets which are then blended with the natural tobacco. The altered physical structure modifies the combustion process. Furthermore, 'tars' and nicotine can be extracted during preparation of the sheet. The blend may be further manipulated in attempts to reduce the toxicity of the smoke. Puffing or expanding (by air or CO_2) diminishes the tobacco content, and also increases the rate of combustion. Freeze-drying selectively reduces the nicotine and phenol content of the blend (National Cancer Institute, 1977).

Materials added to cigarettes include 'casing' solutions (sugar, syrups, honey, liquorice, chocolate and balsams), humectants (glycerol and glycols) and alcohol soluble flavouring agents (menthol, peppermint, cloves, cinnamon and the like). Many of these additives increase the undesirability of tobacco smoke. For example, liquorice can serve as a precursor of polyaromatic hydrocarbons, while the casing sugars increase the yield of furfural, nicotine and tar.

The cigarette wrapper is usually made from flax paper. It may be impregnated with one or more chemicals to regulate its speed of burning. In some countries the tobacco is wrapped in tobacco leaf, banana leaf, rice paper or parchment paper.

Cigars

Cigar tobacco is always aged and fermented and it thus contains less protein, alkaloids and sugar than cigarette tobacco. The other main distinguishing feature of a cigar is that it is wrapped in a tobacco leaf rather than in paper. Filler, binder and wrapper tobacco are normally air-cured, although reconstituted tobacco is now sometimes used for binder or wrapper.

The concentration of phenols and of aromatic hydrocarbons is similar in cigarette and in cigar smoke (Osman & Barson, 1964; Osman *et al.*, 1963). The nicotine content of particulate matter is also similar for the two types of smoke (Hoffmann *et al.*, 1963), although the nicotine yield per gram of tobacco burnt is 20–40% smaller with a cigar than with a cigarette (Schmetlz *et al.*, 1976). On the other hand, the condensate from cigars contains more benz (α) pyrene and pyridine (Hoffmann *et al.*, 1963; Kuhn, 1966). The smoke of cigars and 'little cigars' also has a substantially higher concentration of carbon monoxide than that from a pipe or cigarette, probably because the tightly rolled leaves in a cigar burn less readily (Wahl, 1899; Armstrong, 1922; Harke, 1970; Hoffmann & Wynder, 1972; Brunnemann & Hoffmann, 1974). Moreover, the carbon monoxide of cigar smoke is unprotonated and is thus readily absorbed by the body (Armitage & Turner, 1970).

Pipe Tobacco

The percentage of US males over the age of 21 years who smoke a pipe decreased from 18.7% in 1964 to 12.4% in 1975 (US National Clearing House for Smoking and Health, 1976). The usual pipe tobacco is made largely from the Burley variety, but some blends also contain mid-rib parts of the plant, crushed between rollers. There may be up to 30% of additives, including 'sauces', casing material such as liquorice that bind the leaf together, sugar and various flavouring agents (Wynder & Hoffmann, 1967).

The pipe-smoker transfers a high proportion of the humectants (and resultant acetone and acetaldehyde) to the inhaled smoke. Combustion

Table 2.1: A Comparison of 'Sidestream' and 'Mainstream' Smoke
(Ratio of Concentrations)

Component	Ratio (sidestream/mainstream)
Hydrogen cyanide	0.03 (0.25)[a]
Acetic acid	0.42
Acetamide	0.68
Total particulates	0.7
Acetylene	0.8
Carbon monoxide	1.3–3.0 (4.6)
'Tar'	1.7[b]
Benzene	1.9
Methyl chloride	2.1
3-4 benzo (α) pyrene	2.1 (3.4)
Phenol	2.1 (2.6)
Aldehydes (total)	2.2
Acetonitrile	2.3 (3.9)
Nicotine	2.5 (1.8–2.8)
Toluene	3.5 (5.6)
Pyrene	3.6
Nitrous oxide, other oxides of nitrogen	3.6
Cadmium	3.6
Carbon dioxide	3.8–10.0
Myosmine	7.0
Pyrrole	7.1
Pyridine	9.5 (10)
Nitrosamines	10–40 (52)
3-vinyl pyridene	16.0 (28)
Naphthalene	16.0
Aniline	30.0
Ammonia	98.0

Notes: a. Alternative values proposed by other authors are shown in parenthesis.
　　　 b. Higher for low tar filter cigarettes.
Source: Based on data collected by Hoegg, 1972; Wakeham, 1972; Brunnemann
et al., 1977a,b).

of the casing materials also increases the yield of furfural, nicotine and
tar.

Effect on Smoke Composition

The toxic chemicals produced by combustion of cigarette, cigar and
pipe tobacco reflect differences in the nature of the tobacco and also
differences in the combustion process (Table 2.1; for example, the
production of benzo (α) pyrene per 100 g of tobacco averages 0.9 μg
for a typical cigarette, 3.4 μg for a typical cigar and 8.5 μg for a typical

pipe; Falk, 1977). Even larger differences are observed for pyrene and anthracene (Campbell & Lindsey, 1957), while respective yields of phenol per 100 g of tobacco are 10 mg for cigars, 25 mg for cigarettes and 69 mg for pipes (Hoffmann *et al.*, 1963).

Mainstream and Sidestream Smoke

When a cigarette is smoked, the atmosphere becomes contaminated by both mainstream and sidestream smoke. The mainstream smoke is inhaled by the smoker and then exhaled into the air. Sidestream smoke (Bogen, 1929) comprises about 95% of the remaining contamination (Lipp, 1965). It is emitted from the burning cone of the cigarette between 'puffs'. 'Smoulder stream' smoke (Hoegg, 1972) emerges from the butt end between 'puffs'. Other small fractions include the 'glow-stream' (emitted by the glowing cone during 'puffs'), the 'effusion stream' escaping along the length of the paper during 'puffs' and the 'diffusion stream' escaping through the paper between 'puffs'.

Mainstream Smoke

The figures normally cited for the composition of mainstream smoke are based upon the use of standard smoking machines (Chapter 1). Such data are reasonably representative of the conditions to which many smokers expose themselves. However, the exposure of the 'passive smoker' varies with the proportion of the toxic materials retained by the smoker, or (in the case of the fetus) the proportion of retained toxins that is transmitted across the placenta. Other variables include the number of 'puffs' taken from a cigarette, and (except for the fetus) the proximity of the smoker in relation to ventilation for dispersion or removal of the smoke.

Baumberger (1923) noted that 48 to 78% of the smoke mass was retained during oral 'puffing', and that retention increased to 74 to 99% when the smoke was inhaled. Similar results were obtained by Greenberg *et al.* (1952) and Mitchell (1962). Dalhamn and his associates examined the retention of individual constituents. If a 'puff' of smoke was held in the mouth for two seconds, there was a substantial retention of water soluble compounds (acetonitrile, 74%; acetaldehyde, 60%; acetone, 56%), but a lesser retention of toluene, 29%, ioprene, 20%, particulate matter, 16% and carbon monoxide, 3% (Dalhamn *et al.*, 1968a). If the smoke was inhaled, the lungs retained 86 to 99% of the volatile substances and particulate matter, and about 54% of the carbon

Figure 2.1: The Aging of Cigarette Smoke

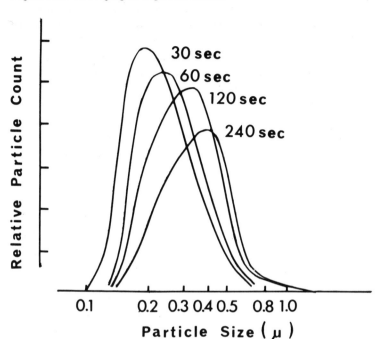

Source: After Keith & Derrick, 1960.

monoxide (Dalhamn *et al.*, 1968b). The smoker normally expels unabsorbed matter through the lips, but further filtration is likely if the smoke is exhaled through the nose.

Sidestream Smoke

The combustion of a typical cigarette involves perhaps ten 2-second 'puffs' and 550 seconds of sidestream combustion. Because the rate of combustion is much faster during 'puffing', about 46% of the tobacco is burnt during the 'puff' phase (Hoegg, 1972).

The physical and chemical characteristics of mainstream and sidestream smoke differ quite widely from each other. The mainstream smoke contains about 5×10^9 particles or droplets per ml. These range in size from less than 0.1 to 1.0 μ, with a mode of around 0.2 μ (Keith & Derrick, 1960; Green & Lane, 1964). The major part of this particulate burden is retained in the lungs of the smoker. Individual particles grow within the respiratory tract, so that the exhaled matter is larger and more heterogenous in size than that inspired from the cigarette butt. The particle size of sidestream smoke that is 60 seconds old ranges from 0.08 to 1.0 μ, with a mode of about 0.15 μ. Some 6.3 $\times$ 10^9 particles are generated by a cigarette with every second of free burning (Keith & Derrick, 1960). The 'aging' of cigarette smoke needs further study. Over the first few minutes, Keith & Derrick (1960) observed a 33% decrease of particle count, with an increase of modal diameter to 0.4 μ (Figure 2.1).

Concentrations of chemicals in the sidestream smoke range from 0.03 to 98 times the mainstream figure (Table 2.1) (Pascasio *et al.*, 1966; Scassellati Sforzolini & Savino, 1968; Bridge & Corn, 1972; Hoegg, 1972; Wakeham, 1972). For some reason as yet unexplained, the sidestream concentration of NO_x is higher for filter than for non-filter cigarettes (Pascasio *et al.*, 1966). If the cigarettes are moist, the mainstream content of both phenol and nicotine diminishes, while the concentration of these two substances in the sidestream smoke increases (Neurath *et al.*, 1964).

Cigar and Pipe Smoke

There has been little formal study of air contamination from cigar and pipe smoke. However, it is known that most users hold the smoke in their mouths without inhaling. The mainstream smoke is thus likely to be exhaled into the atmosphere with relatively little modification.

3 OBSERVED POLLUTION DUE TO CIGARETTE SMOKE ACCUMULATION

In this chapter, we shall examine evidence that cigarette smoking gives rise to significant levels of pollution, discussing data obtained from analysis of contaminated atmospheres (carbon monoxide, nicotine, particulates and other substances) and from the responses of the body to such pollution (blood carboxyhaemoglobin, serum and urinary nicotine and salivary thiocyanate).

Atmospheric Analyses

Exposure of the non-smoker to the toxic constituents of cigarette smoke depends not only on the number of cigarettes that have been smoked, but also on the volume of the room, the efficiency of ventilation, local obstructions to ventilation and the proximity of those who are smoking (Lawther & Commins, 1970; Dublin, 1972; US Surgeon General, 1972; Burns, 1977).

Carbon Monoxide

Carbon monoxide is probably the most frequently determined smoke constituent (Table 3.1). This reflects not only its potential toxicity, but also the ease with which it can be determined by infra-red analysers and portable electro-chemical detectors.

The currently permitted maximum concentrations of carbon monoxide for 8-hour exposure periods are 50 ppm for industrial situations (Shephard, 1981a), and 9 ppm (USA) or 13 ppm (Canada) for the general urban environment (Shephard, 1981b).

The earliest study of CO accumulation due to tobacco smoke was undertaken by Wahl (1899). He machine-smoked 20 cigars in a sealed room of 66 m^3 capacity and reported the resultant CO-concentration as 156 ppm. Normally, the smoker retains a part of the CO that he produces. Baumberger (1923) estimated that 48 to 74% of the CO formed during the 'puffing' of a cigarette was retained by the body. Baumberger ignored both 'burning point' smoke and the possibility of inhalation, and calculated that if ten people were smoking continuously in a room of 27 m^3 capacity, the CO concentration would reach 210 ppm.

Table 3.1: Carbon Monoxide Concentration Observed Under Experimental (E) and 'Real-life' (R) Accumulations of Cigarette Smoke

Location and size	Ventilation (air changes per hour)	CO concentration (ppm)	Author
Room 27 m³ (E)	Closed	210	Baumberger (1923)
House 50 m³ (E)	Closed	7.5	DeRouane & Verduyn (1974)
Room 57 m³ (E)	Closed	50	Harke (1970)
Room 170 m³ (E)	Closed	30–50	Harke (1970)
Room 98 m³ (E)	Closed	80	Harmsen & Effenberger (1957)
Room 25 m³ (E)	Closed	69.8	Hoegg (1972)
Room 30 m³ (E)	Closed	50	Jermini et al. (1976)
Room 14.6 m³ (E)	Closed	24	Pimm et al. (1978)
Room 45 m³ (E)	Closed	38	Russell et al. (1973)
Room 37.5 m³ (E)	Closed	30	Seppänen (1977a)
Room 30 m³ (E)	Closed	24	Weber et al. (1976a,b)
			Weber-Tschopp et al. (1976a,b)
Room 15 m³ (E)	1.0	20	Lawther & Commins (1970)
Room 170 m³ (E)	2.4	8	Harke (1970)
Room 80 m³ (E)	6.4	4.5	Anderson & Dalhamn (1973)
Room 145 m³ (R)	7.0	7.0	Bridge & Corn (1972)
Room 101 m³ (R)	10.6	9.0	Bridge & Corn (1972)
Room 138 m³ (E)	12.0	32.5?	Dublin (1972)
Offices (R)	—	2.5	Chappell & Parker (1977)
Room 78 m³ (R)	—	15.6	Harke (1970)
Offices (R)	—	2.7	Szadkowski et al. (1976)
Conference room (R)	6–8	8–10	Slavin & Hertz (1975)

Table 3.1 Continued

Restaurants and taverns (R)	—	4–13	Chappell & Parker (1977)
Taverns (R)	0–6	13–17	Cuddeback et al. (1976)
Restaurants and taverns (R)	—	8–38	Sebben et al. (1977)
Restaurants (R)	—	< 10	Bonham (1973)
Automobile (E)	Closed	90	Srch (1967)
Automobile (R)	Closed → Open	12 → 23	Harke & Peters (1974)
Inter-city bus (R)	15	18–33	Seiff (1973)
Airport bus (R)	—	6.5–12	Sebben et al. (1977)
Train (R)	—	7	Sebben et al. (1977)
Airplane (R)	15–20	2–5	Fed. Aviat. Admin. (1971)
Ferry (R)	—	18	Godin et al. (1972)
Submarine 66m³ (R)	Yes	40	Cano et al. (1970)
Theatre (R)	—	3.4	Godin et al. (1972)

Source: Based partly on information accumulated by US Surgeon General, 1979.

Bogen (1929) commented that much depended upon the pattern of smoking that was adopted. If small, intermittent 'puffs' were taken, the mainstream smoke contained only 3 ml of carbon monoxide, but with 'fast and furious' smoking, up to 16 ml of CO might be generated. Sidestream smoke had a more stable yield of CO (8 ml with no suction, 12 ml with intermittent or continuous suction on the cigarette).

Hoegg (1972) demonstrated that when 24 cigarettes were smoked simultaneously in a 25 m³ room, the CO concentration attained a peak of 69.8 ppm. Likewise, Jermini *et al.* (1976) noted that the machine-smoking of 20 cigarettes was sufficient to generate the industrial 'maximum acceptable concentration' (MAC) of CO (50 ppm) within a 30 m³ room. Other investigators have also found high CO readings in small and poorly ventilated spaces (Hess, 1971; Lightfoot, 1972). Srch (1967) observed two smokers and two non-smokers in a closed and stationary car. Ten cigarettes were smoked over 60 minutes; the CO level rose to 60 ppm after 20 minutes, and 80 ppm after 60 minutes. Harke *et al.* (1974) and Harke & Peters (1974), reported that when nine cigarettes were smoked inside a small European car a CO concentration of 110 ppm was developed. However, if the car was ventilated, the concentration quickly dropped to 10–20 ppm. The smoking of two cigarettes was sufficient to produce a CO level of 21 ppm under typical driving conditions. Normal ambient air levels were restored within 2–3 minutes of ceasing to smoke.

Much lower CO readings have been observed under most 'real life' conditions (Table 3.1). Bridge and Corn (1972) measured CO concentrations at two domestic parties where about 50% of the group were smokers. About 60 cigarettes and 15 cigars were consumed over 1.5 hours, but the CO concentration was only 7–9 ppm. Harke (1970) and Harke *et al.* (1972) had a subject smoke 11 cigarettes over five hours in a 30 m³ room, and again the CO level remained below 10 ppm. Anderson & Dalhamn (1973) observed that seven smokers consumed 37 cigarettes, nine small cigars and four pipes when they sat in an 80 m³ room for two hours. The ventilation rate was only six air changes per hour but, nevertheless, the CO concentration did not rise above 4.5 ppm. The extent of CO accumulation seems critically dependent upon ventilation of the room or other closed space (Figure 3.1). Jones & Fagan (1974) based their calculation on a 85 m³ room, occupied by 25 smokers; they assumed that each smoker would consume four cigarettes per hour, liberating 74 mg of CO per cigarette. On this basis, two air changes per hour (a ventilation of 2.8 m³ min⁻¹) was sufficient to keep CO concentrations below the MAC (50 ppm), but a much greater

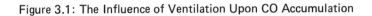

Figure 3.1: The Influence of Ventilation Upon CO Accumulation

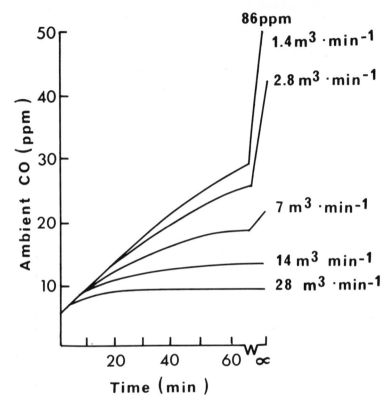

Source: Based on data from Jones & Fagan, 1974, for room of 85 m³ capacity, occupied by 25 smokers.

ventilation (28 m³ min⁻¹, 20 air changes per hour) was needed to meet the US air quality criterion of 9 ppm. Nevertheless, these calculations assumed both a high occupancy for the room and a high rate of cigarette consumption by the inmates.

Smoky offices are a practical concern of many non-smokers, since the polluted atmosphere must be endured for up to eight hours per day. Worse conditions are encountered in many bars and restaurants, particularly if the owners economise on heating or refrigeration by recirculating stale air. Sebben *et al.* (1977) attributed much of the observed range of CO levels (8 to 38 ppm) to differences of occupancy and ventilation, although further factors in some restaurants and bars were carbon monoxide generated by grills and barbecues, and proximity to automobile exhaust from densely travelled streets. The average indoor and outdoor CO concentrations found by Sebben *et al.* (1977) were 14.1 and 9.1 ppm respectively. The important contribution of cigarette smoking to this gradient was indicated by the rise of indoor concentrations from an average of 8.7 ppm when the bars opened at 6 pm to a more constant plateau of 14 to 15 ppm between 7 pm and midnight; by way of contrast, outdoor CO concentrations fell steadily over the evening period. For many people, patronage of a smoke-filled bar is a matter of personal choice, but the employees (bar-tenders, dancers and waitresses) are obliged to withstand such atmospheres for up to eight hours per day, while carrying out moderately heavy physical work. Unfortunately, most of those employed in the catering industry are minimum wage staff and there is no provision for the medical screening of those who are particularly vulnerable to CO exposure.

A third area where non-smokers frequently make complaint about the accumulation of tobacco smoke is in public service vehicles. Available information (Federal Aviation Administration, 1971; Godin *et al.*, 1972; Seiff, 1973; Sebben *et al.*, 1977) shows surprisingly low readings in all such vehicles except a very crowded ferry boat (Godin *et al.*, 1972) and an inter-city bus (Seiff, 1973). On the latter, a blower system supposedly provided 15 air changes per hour. Under the worst possible conditions (fully loaded, 50% of the passengers smoking all of the time), the CO level reached 33 ppm, compared with 7 ppm outside the vehicle. In the 'realistic worst case' (rear 20% of coach occupied by individuals smoking 50% of the time), CO concentrations were 18 ppm inside and 13 ppm outside the vehicle. The Federal Aviation Administration (1971) collected samples on both military and commercial aircraft; air was drawn from the breathing zone of each passenger, outside the zone of turbulence created by the over-seat ventilation system. Carbon monoxide readings were typically < 2 ppm, and in only one sample did the CO concentration exceed 5 ppm.

In view of the careful sampling adopted, it is difficult to argue that the readings were unrepresentative of the conditions encountered by the passengers, although some trapping of still and unpolluted air is probably caused by the high-backed seats used in buses and planes.

Nicotine

The current threshold limit for industrial exposure to nicotine is a concentration of 0.5 mg·m^{-3} (American Conference of Government

Table 3.2: Nicotine Concentrations Observed During Experimental (E) and 'Real-life' (R) Accumulations of Cigarette Smoke

Location and size	Ventilation (air changes per hour)	Nicotine Concentration (mg·m⁻³)	Author
Room 38 m³ (E)	None	.51	Harke *et al.* (1972)
Room 57 m³ (E)	None	.56	Harke (1970)
Room 98 m³ (E)	None	5.20	Harmsen & Effenberger (1957)
Room 170 m³ (E)	None	.72	Harke (1970)
Room 170 m³ (E)	2.4	.10	Harke (1970)
Room 80 m³ (E)	6.4	.38	Anderson & Dalhamn (1973)
Room 57 m³ (E)	7.2	.12	Harke (1970)
Restaurant/tavern (R)	—	0.003–0.010	Hinds & First (1975)
Bus (R)	—	0.006	Hinds & First (1975)
Train (R)	—	0.005	Hinds & First (1975)
Submarine 66 m³ (R)	Yes	0.032	Cano *et al.* (1970)

Source: Based partly on information accumulated by US Surgeon General, 1979.

Industrial Hygienists, 1974). This figure is sometimes exceeded, particularly under experimental conditions (where a substantial number of cigarettes have been burnt in small and poorly ventilated rooms).

Harmsen & Effenberger (1957) noted that a reading of 5.2 mg·m⁻³ was associated with a carbon monoxide concentration of 80 ppm (Table 3.2). Several other authors have encountered nicotine readings in the range of 0.4-0.6 mg·m⁻³. However, levels are much lower (0.003-0.030 mg·m⁻³) in 'real life' situations where adequate ventilation is available. In the worst reported 'real-life' situation (a submarine, 0.030 mg·m⁻³) the non-smokers were exposed for 24 hours per day (Cano *et al.*, 1970). During this time they inspired approximately 15 m³ of air, so that in terms of nicotine dosage, they inhaled the equivalent of 0.5 medium nicotine, or six low nicotine cigarettes per day.

Particulate Matter

Particulate counts (Table 3.3) are a little difficult to interpret unless control observations are obtained, since tobacco smoke is not a unique source of atmospheric particles. On the other hand, it has been long recognized that the indoor 'suspended particulate' readings obtained from such devices as a Hemeon smoke stain indicator depend largely upon the smoking habits of the inhabitants of a building (Shephard *et al.*, 1958). Further, there is a significant leftward shift of the particle

Table 3.3: Concentration of Particulate Matter Observed During Experimental (E) and 'Real-life' (R) Accumulation of Cigarette Smoke

Location and size	Ventilation (air changes per hour)	Particulate matter ($mg \cdot m^{-3}$)	Author
Room 25 m³ (E)	None	17	Hoegg (1972)
Room 15 m³ (E)	1	3	Lawther & Commins (1970)
Home 425 m³ (E)	0.5	2.7	McNall (1975)
(E)	3	1.1	McNall (1975)
Tavern (R)	0	0.98	Cuddeback *et al.* (1976)
	6	0.33	Cuddeback *et al.* (1976)
Aircraft (R)	15–20	< 0.12	Fed. Aviat. Admin. (1971)
Room 145 m³ (R)	7.0	2.8–4.3	Bridge & Corn (1972)
Room 101 m³ (R)	10.6	2.1–3.2	Bridge & Corn (1972)

Source: Based partly on information accumulated by US Surgeon General, 1979.

size distribution curve when a room is occupied by a smoker (Kensler, 1960; Figure 3.2). Harmsen & Effenberger (1957) used a conifuge to compare the airborne particulate concentration in smoking and non-smoking compartments of a railway carriage; particle concentrations were four times higher in the smoking compartment. Bridge & Corn (1972) collected samples at two domestic parties where about 60 cigarettes and 15 cigars had been consumed over 1.5 hours; suspended particulate readings reached the levels encountered in fairly dusty industrial situations (up to 4.3 $mg \cdot m^{-3}$).

Particulate readings are of concern to the non-smoker on two counts: (i) the particulate burden is not being reduced appreciably by current modifications in cigarette design; and (ii) the particulate phase contains many of the very toxic constituents of tobacco smoke, including most of the carcinogens. Unfortunately, it is difficult to infer particulate concentrations from measurements of gas phase pollutants such as carbon monoxide, since the air gradually clears of particulate matter through aggregation, impaction and deposition of the individual particles.

Other Pollutants

Galuskinová (1964) reported that the concentration of the known carcinogen benzo (α) pyrene ranged from 28–144 $ng \cdot m^{-3}$ in a smoke-filled restaurant. However, part of the pollution observed by Galuskinová could have arisen from cooking. A second study in well-ventilated military and civil aircraft (Federal Aviation Administration, 1971)

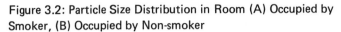

Figure 3.2: Particle Size Distribution in Room (A) Occupied by Smoker, (B) Occupied by Non-smoker

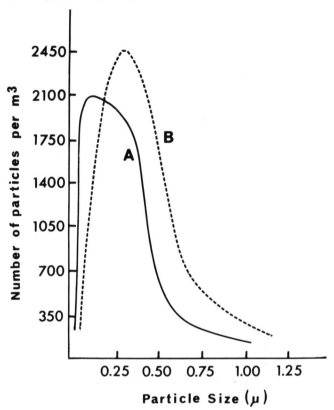

Source: Based on data obtained by Shephard *et al.*, 1958.

failed to observe any readings higher than a fraction of a microgram per m³. Grimmer (research in progress, 1980) noted room concentrations of benz (α) pyrene averaging 22 ng·m⁻³ when five cigarettes per hour were smoked in a 36 m³ room; there was one air change per hour and the CO concentration in these experiments was only about 10 ppm. Having regard to the normal environmental contamination (5–68 ng·m⁻³, depending upon season), Grimmer *et al.* (1977) estimated that passive smoking increased the body burden of polycyclic aromatic hydrocarbons by about 20%.

Dimethylnitrosamine is another potent carcinogen, with an industrial threshold limit of zero ('contact by any route should not be permitted').

Table 3.4: Concentrations of Various Chemicals Observed During Experimental (E) and 'Real-life' (R) Accumulations of Cigarette Smoke

Location and size	Ventilation (air changes (per hour)	Chemical	Concentration ng · l^{-1}	Author
Room 20 m³ (E)	None–Some	Dimethylnitrosamine	0.23–0.33	Brunnemann et al. (1977 a, b)
Train (bar) (R)	–	Dimethylnitrosamine	0.11–0.13	Brunnemann & Hoffmann (1974)
Bar (R)	–	Dimethylnitrosamine	0.24	Brunnemann & Hoffmann (1974)
Room 38 m³ (E)	None	Acetaldehyde	650	Harke (1970)
	None	Acrolein	460	Harke (1970)
Room 170 m³ (E)	None	Acetaldehyde	530	Harke (1970)
	None	Acrolein	390	Harke (1970)
	2.4	Acetaldehyde	500	Harke (1970)
	2.4	Acrolein	40	Harke (1970)
Room 30 m³ (E)	None	Acrolein	950	Jermini et al. (1976)
Room 30 m³ (E)	None	Acetaldehyde	616	Weber et al. (1976a, b)
		Acrolein	275	Weber et al. (1976a, b)
Restaurant (R)	–	Benzopyrene	0.03–0.14	Galuskinova (1964)
Aircraft (R)	15	Benzopyrene	≪ .1	Fed. Aviat. Admin. (1971)

Source: Based partly on information accumulated by US Surgeon General, 1979.

Heavy experimental smoking in an unventilated room yielded concentrations of 0.23 to 2.7 μg$\cdot$m^{-3}, while under 'real-life' conditions readings of 0.11 to 0.24 μg$\cdot$m^{-3} were seen in the bar car of a train, and in a bar (Brunnemann *et al.*, 1977a, b). Because the nitrosamines occur mainly in sidestream smoke, the non-smoker can inhale the mainstream equivalent of 0.5 to 30 cigarettes per day if he or she works in a smoky atmosphere (Brunnemann *et al.*, 1977a, b).

Acrolein and aldehyde levels (Table 3.4) provide an index of the irritant vapours that accumulate from cigarette smoking. The industrially permitted TLV of acrolein (0.1 ppm, 0.25 mg$\cdot$m^{-3}) is exceeded, but only under experimental conditions where a large number of cigarettes have been burnt in a closed room (Harke, 1970; Weber *et al.*, 1976a,b).

Conclusion

In most of the instances discussed, contamination due to cigarette smoke accumulation becomes a health concern only when ventilation is poor or non-existent. However, there is need for further research on the build-up of benz (α) pyrene and dimethylnitrosamine; significant amounts of these very dangerous substances can apparently accumulate in 'real-life' situations.

Body Responses to Pollutants

Epidemiological techniques that have been suggested for estimating exposure to cigarette smoke include determinations of blood carboxyhaemoglobin, measurement of serum nicotine levels and estimates of thiocyanate in plasma, saliva and urine.

Blood Carboxyhaemoglobin

Carbon monoxide accumulates in the body as the pigment carboxyhaemoglobin. Although there are other sources of carbon monoxide than cigarette smoke, the stability of the pigment (half-time of elimination about four hours) makes it a useful indicator of a passive smoke exposure. Determinations can be made upon capillary blood samples, using a spectrophotometer (Commins & Lawther, 1965; Maas *et al.*, 1970; Commins, 1975). Alternatively, the carbon monoxide concentration may be examined in expired or alveolar gas (Sjöstrand, 1948; Dahlström, 1955; Jones *et al.*, 1958; Henderson & Apthorp, 1960; Hackney *et al.*, 1962; McIlvaine *et al.*, 1969).

The first determination of blood COHb% increments during

passive smoking was carried out by Srch (1967). Two non-smokers sat in a stationary car along with two chain smokers. The CO level within the car reached 60 ppm in 20 minutes, and then climbed more slowly to a final figure of 80 ppm at the end of the one hour exposure period. The final COHb of the non-smokers was a substantial 5%.

In the experiments of Harke (1970) and Harke & Bleichert (1972), 105 cigarettes were smoked in an unventilated room over the course of two hours. The blood COHb of non-smokers occupying the room increased from 0.9 to 2.1% during this period. When a similar number of cigarettes were consumed with adequate ventilation, the CO concentration was much lower (5 ppm), although even in the latter circumstances the COHb of the non-smokers was said to have increased from 1.1 to 1.6%. Nevertheless, no changes of skin temperature, blood pressure or pulse rate were seen when the subjects occupied a room where as many as 150 cigarettes were machine-smoked over the course of 30 minutes.

Russell *et al.* (1973, 1975) brought the CO concentration in a small room to 38 ppm through a combination of actual smoking and the smouldering of cigarettes in ash-trays. Over 78 minutes of exposure to this atmosphere, the blood COHb of twelve non-smokers increased from 1.6 to 2.6%, equivalent to the effect of smoking nine cigarettes. Nevertheless, almost all subjects found the conditions very unpleasant, with more smoke accumulation than they encountered during normal living. Anderson & Dalhamn (1973) made their observations under 'real-life' conditions of ventilation and smoking; they found no increase in the blood COHb of five non-smokers when they shared a room with seven heavy smokers (CO concentration 4.5 ppm). Aronow (1978) had three volunteers smoke 15 cigarettes over the course of two hours. When the ventilation of the room was not in use, the COHb of non-smoking occupants increased from 1.30 to 2.28%; given relatively brisk ventilation (11.4 air changes per hour), the COHb of the non-smokers still rose from 1.26 to 1.77%.

Such observations are sufficient to indicate that passive smoking can increase blood carboxyhaemoglobin levels, particularly when ventilation is poor (Wakeham, 1977). The size of the increment observed depends on: (i) the baseline COHb (0.4% due to endogenous carbon monoxide production, but often 1.0 to 1.5% in an urban environment); (ii) the average ambient CO concentration; (iii) the duration of exposure; and (iv) the ambient oxygen pressure. In most circumstances, the half-time for equilibration with ambient conditions is 3–4 hours (Table 3.5). Furthermore, if a subject has been driving in heavy traffic (up to 50

Table 3.5: The Anticipated Blood COHb Readings Resulting from the Exposure of Healthy Non-smokers to Known CO Concentrations for a Specified Period

Concentration of carbon monoxide (ppm)	Duration of exposure and resulting COHb%					
	15 min	30 min	60 min	3 hours	8 hours	Equilibrium
5	0.4	0.4	0.5	0.6	0.8	0.9
10	0.4	0.5	0.6	1.1	1.7	1.8
20	0.5	0.7	0.9	1.7	3.0	3.5
30	0.6	0.8	1.3	2.4	4.5	5.0
40	0.7	1.0	1.5	2.8	5.9	6.1
50	0.8	1.3	1.9	3.5	7.0	7.8
100	1.4	2.2	3.0	6.5	12.5	14.0

Source: Based on data accumulated by Shephard, 1981a.

Table 3.6: Influence of Physical Activity Upon the Blood COHb% Resulting from Various Exposures of Normal Healthy Non-smoking Adults to Carbon Monoxide

Concentration of carbon monoxide (ppm)	Blood carboxyhaemoglobin level								
	15-min exposure			60-min exposure			8-hour exposure		
	S	M	H	S	M	H	S	M	H
5	0.52	0.54	0.56	0.58	0.63	0.68	0.91	0.91	0.89
10	0.55	0.61	0.67	0.71	0.90	1.10	1.5	1.7	1.7
25	0.66	0.84	1.00	1.1	1.7	2.2	3.3	4.1	4.2
50	0.82	1.20	1.60	1.7	3.0	4.1	6.4	8.0	8.3

S = sedentary; M = moderate activity; H = heavy work.
Source: Based on data developed by WHO, 1979.

ppm CO) and then enters a room moderately polluted by cigarette smoke (25 ppm CO), some elimination of CO will occur (although less rapidly and less completely than would be possible in 'clean' air). Thus Szadkowski *et al.* (1976) found that the blood COHb% of passive smokers in an office-building dropped from 0.82 to 0.63% between 8 am and 3 pm. Physical activity has little effect upon the final equilibrium COHb%, but over shorter periods of exposure a person who is engaged in hard physical work reaches a higher COHb reading than a sedentary subject who is exposed to the same ambient concentration of carbon monoxide (Table 3.6).

Nicotine And Its Metabolites

Nicotine has the significant advantage from an epidemiological point of view that it is unique to tobacco. If nicotine or one of its metabolites is found in the body of a non-smoker, it thus provides an unequivocal proof of passive exposure to tobacco smoke. Nicotine itself is metabolized to cotinine, with a half-life of about an hour (Russell *et al.*, 1977); however, the cotinine persists in the body for several days and can be detected by modern methods of gas chromatography (Hengen & Hengen, 1978).

Cano *et al.* (1970) examined the nicotine excretion of non-smoking sailors living on a submarine. The ambient levels of nicotine (15–32 $\mu g \cdot m^{-3}$) were much lower than those developed in some closed-room experiments; nevertheless, some nicotine was found in the urine, up to 1% of that found in smoking subjects. Harke (1970) tested the urine for both nicotine and cotinine, and he also found an excretion only 1% of that seen in smokers. Russell & Feyerabend (1975) demonstrated nicotine levels of 90 $\mu g \cdot ml^{-1}$ in the plasma and 80 $\mu g \cdot ml^{-1}$ in the urine of non-smokers following 78 minutes exposure to dense cigarette smoke (38 ppm CO); by way of comparison, the average urinary nicotine of the smokers was thirteen times as large (12.4 $\mu g \cdot ml^{-1}$). Horning *et al.* (1973) reported that non-smokers who shared a laboratory with smokers excreted about 5% as much nicotine as that found in the urine of the smokers.

We may conclude that nicotine measurements support the view that passive smokers are forced to inspire some cigarette smoke; biological specimens indicate an exposure similar to that already calculated from the gas phase concentration of nicotine (above), the equivalent of one to two cigarettes, distributed over the course of the day. Such quantities of nicotine are unlikely to have any substantial pharmacological effect in their own right (Russell & Feyerabend, 1975); however, they serve to indicate that the non-smoker is encountering other more dangerous constituents of cigarette smoke.

Thiocyanate

The thiocyanate that is found in biological fluids comes from two main sources — cyanogen-containing vegetables (casava root, cabbage, broccoli, cauliflower, turnips, radishes, garlic, horse-radish, mustard and almonds — Denson *et al.*, 1967), and the hydrogen cyanide of tobacco smoke (Pettigrew & Fell, 1972). Occasionally, there may also be an industrial source, as in a study of electroplating workers (Radojicic, 1973). The absorbed hydrogen cyanide is rapidly converted to thiocyanate by the liver, kidney and intestines. Thiocyanate provides a fairly stable index of exposure since it has a biological half-life of some 14 days (Pettigrew & Fell, 1972). Typical blood levels of thiocyanate are 25 μ mol·l^{-1} in vegetarian non-smokers, 18 μ mol·l^{-1} in non-vegetarian non-smokers and 80 to 100 μ mol·l^{-1} in smokers (Densen *et al.*, 1967; Dastur *et al.*, 1972; Vogt *et al.*, 1977).

Perhaps because of complications introduced by variations of diet, thiocyanate determinations have not yet been applied to the analysis of passive smoking, except during pregnancy (Bottoms *et al.*, research in progress, 1980); the fetus of a smoking mother has a blood thiocyanate level about 80% of that seen in the maternal circulation.

4 CARBON MONOXIDE AND THE BODY

In this chapter, we shall look at certain effects of low concentrations of carbon monoxide upon the human body, and will consider how far such reactions are likely to be encountered in the 'passive smoker'. Topics that will be examined include a deterioration of psychomotor function, a decrease of effort tolerance and an exacerbation of ischaemic heart disease. All are issues that have received extensive discussion in the context of urban and industrial air pollution (Shephard, 1981a, b). We shall also examine specific circumstances that increase sensitivity to carbon monoxide.

Deterioration of Psychomotor Function

The psychomotor effects of small doses of carbon monoxide reflect the development of oxygen lack within the central nervous system. One factor contributing to this phenomenon is the firm binding of carbon monoxide to the haemoglobin pigment, but a more important explanation is probably a leftward displacement of the oxygen dissociation curve of haemoglobin which occurs following exposure to carbon monoxide. The leftward shift increases the proportion of oxygen that remains bound to haemoglobin in tissues with a low partial pressure of oxygen, and inevitably local manifestations of hypoxia become more likely.

In animals, a 2% increase of blood carboxyhaemoglobin (COHb%) is sufficient to reduce tissue oxygen pressures within the brain (Zorn, 1972). However, there is still considerable controversy concerning the minimum COHb% necessary to cause a derangement of psychomotor function in man. Problems of investigation include: (i) a lack of precision in many psychomotor tests; (ii) the prolonged learning schedules needed for valid use of the more complicated and sensitive tests; (iii) a substantial reserve of mental function, normally untapped but available during hypoxia; (iv) changes of cerebral arousal that often develop over prolonged experiments; and (v) possible physiological adaptations to carbon monoxide poisoning (including an increased oxygen delivery through the cerebral blood vessels).

Some authors have found no deterioration of central nervous function

Table 4.1: Some Reported Effects of Carbon Monoxide Upon Central
Nervous Function, with the Corresponding Blood Carboxyhaemoglobin
Readings

Function	Blood COHb%	Author
Vigilance task	1.8	Beard & Grandstaff (1972)
Errors of time-estimation	1.8	Beard & Grandstaff (1972)
Vigilance task	2.3–3.1	Fodor & Winneke (1972)
Vigilance task	?3.0	Groll-Knapp *et al.* (1972)
Auditory duration discrimination	2.5–4.0	Beard & Wertheim (1967)
Visual intensity discrimination	3.0	Beard & Grandstaff (1970)
Tracking task	3.0	Mikulka *et al.* (1970)
Choice reaction time	3.5–4.0	Ramsey (1972)
Visual acuity	4.5	McFarland *et al.* (1944)
Vigilance	5.0	Horvath *et al.* (1971)
Mental performance and finger dexterity	7.2	Bender *et al.* (1971)

even at very high COHb levels. Thus Forbes *et al.* (1937) reported no change of reaction time, binocular vision and eye-hand co-ordination despite a COHb of 30%. Likewise, Stewart *et al.* (1970) found no alteration of hand and foot 'reaction times', hand-steadiness, manual dexterity, visual acuity, depth perception or time estimation at a COHb of 11–13%, while O'Donnell *et al.* (1971) detected no changes of critical flicker-fusion frequency, time estimation or mental arithmetic ability with COHb readings of up to 12.7%.

Other investigators have found a disturbance of function with a COHb of only 1.8 to 5.0% (Table 4.1). They attribute previous reports of a much higher threshold to: (i) a lack of tests at low doses of CO; and (ii) a sample size that was insufficient to allow for variability in the test methodology. The earliest detectable effect of CO is some deterioration of vigilance, such as failure to detect a difference in signal length (Beard & Wertheim, 1967; Beard & Grandstaff, 1972), tone loudness (Groll-Knapp *et al.*, 1972) or light brightness (McFarland *et al.*, 1944; Halperin *et al.*, 1959; Beard & Grandstaff, 1970; Horvath *et al.*, 1971). Another early manifestation of CO poisoning is difficulty in time estimation. Such conclusions are in keeping with the effects of high altitude hypoxia as observed during and immediately following World War II.

While many authors are prepared to accept that there is some CO-induced deterioration of psychomotor function at a blood COHb of

3 to 4%, the basis for the worsening of auditory duration discrimination reported by Beard & Wertheim (1967) remains more controversial. COHb was not determined in the Beard & Wertheim experiments, but a final figure of 2 to 3% COHb was deduced from the CO concentration within the exposure chamber (55 ppm) and the exposure time (2½ hours). Attempts to replicate their results have been generally unsuccessful (O'Donnell *et al.*, 1970; Stewart *et al.*, 1970; Weir *et al.*, 1973; Otto *et al.*, 1979; Wright & Shephard, 1978), although Beard & Grandstaff (1972) have presented further evidence of functional disturbances including an impairment of time estimation at COHb readings of 2 to 3%. Critics of Beard & Wertheim (1967) have suggested that their findings were obtained mainly because arousal of the subjects had been artificially reduced; certainly, participants in their tests were confined to a small audiometric booth throughout a lengthy exposure to carbon monoxide. The extent of arousal is plainly a fundamental issue when interpreting vigilance tests. Nevertheless, it can be argued that a rather boring task carried out in an audiometric booth bears some similarity to the usual demands of highway driving (a situation where CO can accumulate from both smoking and vehicle exhaust).

In at least two of the experiments cited in Table 4.1, the initial disturbance of psychomotor function was corrected as the experiment continued (Beard & Grandstaff, 1972; Fodor & Winneke, 1972). This suggests the possibility of physiological compensation, whether by a greater use of the existing cerebral reserve, an increase of arousal or an augmentation of cerebral blood flow.

The immediate disturbances of cerebral function induced by CO-exposure are physiological, reversible and hard to detect. However, the loss of skill could have serious practical implications when carrying out certain skilled tasks such as driving a car. Yabroff *et al.* (1974) noted some of the ways in which a vehicle operator might be affected, including: (a) loss of the acoustic and auditory vigilance needed for defensive driving; (b) a deterioration of colour vision that could affect the perception of brake and traffic lights; (c) a worsening of brightness discrimination, affecting distance estimation; (d) a loss of peripheral vision, needed to watch the environment, road signs and other traffic; and (e) a slowing of glare recovery (important in night driving and when emerging from a tunnel).

The assessment of ability to drive a motor vehicle is quite difficult. Some investigators such as Wright *et al.* (1973) have based conclusions upon use of a laboratory driving simulator. The techniques required to operate such a machine differ quite markedly from the skills needed when driving a normal car. The subject is confronted by a film depicting a substantial range of emergencies occurring over a short period of time. However, the situation can be viewed with some detachment, since the operator realises that there is no personal danger in the situation. Furthermore, the normal feedback of information from engine noise and movement of the vehicle is lacking. Wright *et al.* (1973) arbitrarily divided the simulator tasks into two categories — 'automatic' and 'careful' driving habits. The latter underwent a statistically marginal deterioration ($0.1 > P > 0.05$ by χ^2 test) following a 3.4% *increase* of COHb (total COHb 5% in non-smokers). Rummo & Sarlanis (1974) used a simulator that tested responses to slowing of a car immediately ahead. Subjects described the procedure as 'realistic but boring'. Response times were slowed and steering reversals were decreased after a 6 to 8% increase of COHb, but the deterioration of performance was statistically significant only if data for one smoker were excluded.

Experiments conducted while driving actual vehicles have indicated a similar disturbance of function, but only after exposure to quite large doses of CO (Rockwell & Ray, 1967; Ray & Rockwell, 1970; McFarland, 1973; Weir *et al.*, 1973; Rockwell & Weir, 1975). Ray & Rockwell (1970) noted a deterioration of both time and distance estimation, poorer tail-light discrimination and slower determination of velocity changes in the car ahead, the overall result being a decreased ability to control following distance. Weir *et al.* (1973) observed perceptual narrowing at 7 and 12% COHb, the driver spending less time looking outside the immediate forward direction. Other changes were seen at 12% COHb (Weir *et al.*, 1973), including a reduction in the number of glances into the rear-view mirror prior to leap-frog passing, increased variations in vehicle speed, decreased steering movements and delay in the processing of visual information. One important objection to most road tests is that under normal circumstances the required tasks do not demand a full commitment of the subject's cerebral reserve; it is thus possible to compensate for CO poisoning by trying harder. Forbes *et al.* (1937) increased COHb levels by 30%, and then examined reaction times, co-ordination and perception in the context of driving ability. Although the subjects could concentrate for long enough to perform the laboratory tasks quite well, they were subjectively aware that their capacity to operate a vehicle had been impaired.

It is unfortunate that most investigators have found it necessary to conduct roadway tests with very light mental loads. For reasons of safety, tests have usually been carried out at disused airfields or on unopened expressways at relatively low speeds. The subjects have thus found driving very easy, with substantial scope to compensate for any CO induced loss of cerebral function. Nevertheless, a decrease of cerebral reserve could have critical consequences in the event of an emergency. McFarland (1973) had his subjects drive with a movable mask over the face (the technique of 'visual occlusion'). Carbon monoxide exposure (17% COHb) had no effect upon the overt performance in terms of steering-wheel reversals over unit distance, but a diminished cerebral reserve was suggested by the fact that subjects demanded more roadway viewing time.

The frequency of vehicle accidents has yet to be linked convincingly to CO exposure. One major problem in establishing such a relationship is the overwhelming influence of alcohol ingestion upon the incidence of traffic accidents. Yabroff *et al.* (1974) noted that the proportion of accident victims having a COHb over 5% was greater than would have been anticipated in a random sample of the population. However, there are several alternative explanations of the observation: (i) there is known to be an association between alcoholism and cigarette smoking; (ii) accidents may be caused by the mechanical problems of smoking in a fast-moving vehicle (for instance, searching the floor for a dropped cigarette); (iii) accidents may be provoked by constituents of cigarette smoke other than carbon monoxide; (iv) there may be some linkage between the habit of cigarette smoking and an accident-prone personality; and (v) there may be an interaction between alcohol ingestion and CO exposure, so that amounts of either substances which are harmless in themselves could have a disastrous joint effect upon driving skills (Weir *et al.*, 1975).

We may conclude that in the normal, healthy non-smoking adult living at sea-level, it is not possible to demonstrate any deterioration of psychomotor function with a COHb of less than 3 to 4%. Even if CO exposure induces readings of this magnitude, the effects upon the central nervous system are readily countered by physiological mechanisms of adaptation. It has yet to be shown conclusively that the liability to traffic accidents is increased by such doses of carbon monoxide.

Effort Tolerance

The prime determinant of an individual's tolerance of heavy physical work is the maximum oxygen intake, the ability to transport oxygen from the atmosphere to the working tissues (Shephard, 1977, 1978a).

Oxygen transport depends in turn upon the maximum cardiac output, and the oxygen carrying capacity of unit volume of blood.

Since carbon monoxide combines firmly with haemoglobin, displacing oxygen, one might anticipate a linear relationship between any increase of COHb and the resultant decrease of effort tolerance. However, some authors have argued that there is a threshold of COHb, below which no loss of oxygen transport is observed. Such views probably reflect the difficulty in demonstrating a small biological response in the face of experimental variation; certainly there has been no convincing demonstration of a zero intercept on the graph relating COHb% and maximum oxygen intake. Clark & Coburn (1975) have suggested that part of the metabolic response to carbon monoxide exposure arises from a poisoning of intracellular mechanisms for oxygen utilization. However, a strong argument against this view is that the effects of carbon monoxide are rather similar whether it be administered suddenly, as a bolus, or more gradually, through exposure to moderate atmospheric contamination.

One report (Goldsmith, 1970) described a deterioration of competitive swimming times after exposure to a CO concentration of 30 ppm. Unfortunately, COHb% was not determined, and since the CO accumulation was due to vehicle exhaust, other pollutants could have contributed to the observed loss of performance.

Heart rate, respiratory rate and respiratory minute volume during maximum exercise are unchanged by exposure to CO (Ekblom & Huot, 1972; Maugh, 1972; Vogel & Gleser, 1972), but there is a decline of maximum oxygen intake that is approximately proportional to the increase of COHb% (Vogel & Gleser, 1972). Raven *et al.* (1974) and Horvath *et al.* (1975) suggested that the relationship became non-linear at a COHb saturation of less then 6%. Nevertheless, the response that they observed at low COHb readings appears compatible with a linear extrapolation of the data obtained following exposure to large doses of carbon monoxide. The experiments of Horvath *et al.* (1975) were 'double-blind' in design, but nevertheless the subjects were able to identify those tests where large doses of CO had been administered. Under such conditions, the legs felt heavy and the exercise task seemed more difficult.

Quite modest doses of carbon monoxide shorten the endurance time for hard physical work (Seppänen, 1977b; Ekblom & Huot, 1972), Drinkwater *et al.* (1974) and Raven *et al.* (1974) found a statistically significant effect following exposure to a CO concentration of 50 ppm

(5 Pa), despite a very small (2.1%) increase of COHb (total COHb of non-smokers 2.8%).

We may conclude that any unnecessary exposure to carbon monoxide will cause a deterioration of effort tolerance proportional to the increment of COHb. However, the concentrations encountered by the passive smoker are unlikely to have practical importance unless an individual intends to engage in endurance athletics. In such a situation, even a 1% reduction of oxygen transport could represent the difference between victory and defeat.

Exacerbation of Ischaemic Heart Disease

Carbon monoxide exposure has an immediate adverse effect upon patients with manifestations of vascular disease such as angina and intermittent claudication. It may also contribute to the development of atherosclerosis. Ayres *et al.* (1965) studied coronary vascular gas pressures during a 'bolus' exposure to carbon monoxide that produced COHb levels of 6 to 12%. The coronary arteriovenous oxygen difference was widened, both in normal subjects and in patients with pre-existing coronary vascular atherosclerosis, while hypoxia of the heart muscle was indicated by a decreased extraction of lactate from the coronary blood stream. A part of the tissue hypoxia may have arisen from extravascular escape of CO, since a bolus was administered with a very high instantaneous CO concentration (Ayres *et al.*, 1970).

Individuals with a normal coronary circulation were able to compensate partially for the CO exposure through an increase of coronary perfusion, but this type of adaptation was not possible for those with established coronary vascular disease (Ayres *et al.*, 1968, 1969; Adams *et al.*, 1973; Horvath, 1973; Young & Stone, 1976). Because of shifts in the haemoglobin dissociation curve (Figure 4.1), coronary blood flow must be increased some 20% to compensate for a 5% increase of COHb% (Permutt & Farhi, 1969).

Aronow *et al.* (1972) examined the influence of CO exposure upon the time to onset of exercise-induced angina. In their first experiment, patients liable to angina were driven along a Los Angeles freeway in a vehicle with open windows. The ambient CO concentration averaged 53 ppm (5.3 Pa) and, over a 90-minute period of exposure, blood COHb levels increased by 4% to an average of 5.1%. As a result, the endurance of a standard cycle ergometer test diminished from 249 to 174 seconds. The electrocardiogram also showed earlier ST segmental

Figure 4.1: The Influence of Carbon Monoxide Exposure Upon the Shape of the Oxygen Dissociation Curve of Haemoglobin (Schematic)

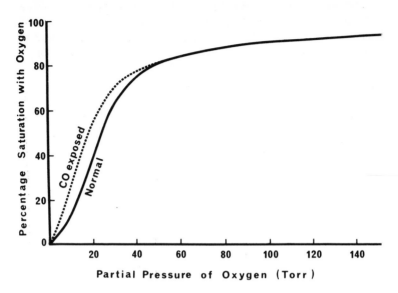

depression; this appeared at a lower than usual systolic blood pressure/ heart rate product, after less work had been performed. On a second occasion, the freeway drive was repeated, but the subject was allowed to breathe CO-free air from a cylinder. The COHb then dropped to 0.65%, and the endurance time on the cycle ergometer was unchanged from the initial control reading.

The two main objections to this experiment were: (i) the exposure was not 'double-blind'; and (ii) any response could have arisen from components of vehicle exhaust other than carbon monoxide (Theodore, 1973). Aronow & Isbell (1973) thus carried out further laboratory studies where subjects inhaled either pure compressed air or air containing carbon monoxide, according to a double-blind protocol. On the days that carbon monoxide was administered, the COHb increased 1.65% (to a total of 2.5-3.0%), but this was sufficient to reduce the time to onset of angina from 224 to 188 seconds. Furthermore, the systolic pressure/heart rate product at the onset of angina was reduced, although no significant electrocardiographic abnormalities were seen in any of the tests.

Anderson *et al.* (1973) had subjects with stable angina breathe air or carbon monoxide (concentration 50 or 100 ppm) for four hours prior to a treadmill walk. In the two experimental conditions (2.9% and 4.5% increase of COHb respectively), the time to onset of angina was reduced rather equally, although the higher concentration of CO produced longer-lasting pain. Jones & Knelson (in preparation) analysed the results of these several experiments and argued that the time to onset of angina was linearly related to the increment of COHb%, with no zero intercept. There was thus no safe minimum dose of CO that would not worsen exercise-induced angina.

Aronow (1974) carried out one experiment with passive smoking, using as subjects patients with angina pectoris. When the room was ventilated, the blood COHb rose to 1.77%, and when there was no ventilation an average COHb of 2.28% was observed. In both circumstances, the time to onset of exercise-induced angina was shortened, by 22% and 38% respectively. The heart rate and blood pressure were also increased; although Aronow attributed this to absorption of nicotine, an emotional reaction to the stress of the smoke-filled room is more likely (Waite, 1978).

A final experiment from Aronow's laboratory tested the double-blind inhalation of carbon monoxide in patients with intermittent claudication (Aronow et al., 1974). The time to the onset of claudicant pain was reduced from 174 to 144 seconds of exercise in response to a 1.69% increase of COHb (total 2.8%).

In a more long-term sense, it has been suggested that carbon monoxide exposure is a factor provoking the development of atherosclerosis (Åstrup, 1969; Birstingl et al., 1970; Kjeldsen et al., 1972; Thomsen & Kjeldsen, 1974; Armitage et al., 1976). However, the possible chronic effects of CO upon the vasculature do not seem to be important in the context of passive smoking. Even if CO has such an effect upon a man eating a normal diet, the threshold COHb is relatively high (20–30% COHb), and falls far outside the range anticipated from passive exposure to cigarette smoke.

Sensitive Populations

The average passive smoker does not seem at great risk from CO accumulation unless ventilation is poor. However, there are special personal and environmental circumstances that increase the sensitivity of some populations.

The sensitivity of the fetus to carbon monoxide is widely recognized, with exposure usually occurring through the consumption of cigarettes by the mother. (This variant of passive smoking is discussed in Chapter 10.) Pregnant women and the newborn also have an increased vulnerability to cigarette smoke.

A substantial segment of the population suffers from various forms of hypoxic disease. Such disease makes an individual more sensitive to carbon monoxide exposure only if it limits the transport of oxygen to those tissues particularly vulnerable to CO poisoning (the brain, the heart and skeletal muscle). One obvious candidate pathology is cerebrovascular disease. There do not seem to have been any formal studies of the CO sensitivity of this population. In contrast, there has been considerable investigation of interactions between coronary atherosclerosis and CO exposure. Possible effects of CO include a shortening of the time to exercise-induced angina (as discussed above), a lowering of the threshold for abnormalities of cardiac rhythm and an increase in the risk of cardiac death. Animal experiments (Thomsen & Kjeldsen, 1974; DeBias *et al.*, 1976) support the concept that CO poisoning predisposes to abnormalities of heart rhythm. In man, also, there is some evidence that minor electrocardiographic abnormalities are worsened if exercise is undertaken after exposure to carbon monoxide (Hackney *et al.*, 1962; Anderson *et al.*, 1971, 1973). On the other hand, there is as yet no evidence that CO exposure increases the frequency or the severity of chest pain in the normal life of a patient with angina, nor is it established that CO shortens life expectancy or causes other complications in such an individual (Coburn, 1977).

Several reports have indicated an association between CO exposure and deaths from myocardial infarction (Table 4.2). Presumably, the mechanism is that CO increases the likelihood of a fatal abnormality of heart rhythm. Some authors have set the threshold for such an effect at a COHb of 2% to 3%, while others have argued that patients face an increased risk of hospitalization and death with a sustained blood COHb of 1.4% at sea level (Cohen *et al.*, 1969) and 0.9% at an altitude of 1500 metres (Kurt *et al.*, 1978). Such reports must be viewed with some scepticism, since: (i) the affected patients may have encountered much larger doses of CO than those observed at isolated sampling stations; and (ii) factors other than CO exposure may have affected population health in polluted areas of the cities studied.

A study of 35 hospitals in greater Los Angeles disclosed no relationship between local CO concentrations and admissions for myocardial infarction (Cohen *et al.*, 1969), but the case fatality rate was related to atmospheric CO in regions of the city that were highly polluted (weekly average > 8 ppm CO > 0.8 Pa). Although this effect could

Table 4.2: Influence of Carbon Monoxide Exposure Upon Cardiac Morbidity

Variable	Threshold concentration of CO (ppm)	Comment	Authors
Case fatality rate	8 (7-day average)	Effect seen in winter – reduced mortality in areas where pollution *low*	Cohen *et al.* (1969)
Excess cardiovascular deaths	20 (24 hour average)	Allowance for season, temperature and oxidants	Hexter & Goldsmith (1971)
Sudden death myocardial infarction, total arteriosclerotic heart disease	4 versus 9 (24 hour average)	No effect *except* higher post-mortem COHb in arteriosclerotic heart deaths (possibly because smokers describe themselves as ex-smokers)	Kuller *et al.* (1975)
Cardiorespiratory complaints in emergency room	5 (24 hour average) 11 (1 hour average)	Altitude 1500 m	Kurt *et al.* (1978)

have arisen from inter-hospital differences in the characteristics of the patients admitted, or local variations in the standard of medical care, it seems significant that the increase of mortality was seen only in the winter, the season when levels of pollution were high. Nevertheless, it remains arguable that some other factor such as a second pollutant was correlated with CO concentrations.

Hexter & Goldsmith (1971) used a sophisticated multiple regression equation to relate the death rate to daily environmental pollution. After allowing for effects of season, temperature and oxidant concentrations, they concluded that a 24-hour average CO concentration of 20 ppm (2.0 Pa) could still give rise to an excess of eleven cardiovascular deaths per day in the Greater Los Angeles area. Even more striking was the report of Kurt *et al.* (1978), who found an increase of cardio-respiratory emergencies when the ambient CO concentration exceeded 5 ppm (24-hour average) or 11 ppm (one-hour average); however, the sensitivity of this population to CO was probably increased by the altitude of the city concerned (about 1500 metres above sea-level).

Against these reports, which suggest an effect upon cardiovascular health at quite modest concentrations of carbon monoxide, Curphey *et al.* (1965) found no relationship between COHb levels and the cause of death in a survey of 2,207 post-mortems conducted in the Los Angeles area. Likewise, Kuller *et al.* (1975) could not detect any 'clustering' of myocardial infarctions or heart attacks on days when the CO concentration around the Johns Hopkins (Baltimore) Hospital was high (9 ppm, compared to 0–4 ppm).

We may conclude that there is some evidence that exposure to CO increases the risk of developing severe or fatal manifestations of ischaemic heart disease, in man as in animals (Goldsmith & Aronow, 1975). However, the threshold concentration may be quite high unless the subject is sensitized by simultaneous exposure to high altitudes. Furthermore, the vulnerable subjects are probably limited to a small proportion of the total populace, particularly those with unstable angina or an acute myocardial infarction.

A wide range of other conditions (various types of hypoxia, increased metabolism, increased endogenous production of carbon monoxide and interactions with other drugs) make subjects more sensitive to an accumulation of carbon monoxide (Table 4.3; Forbes *et al.*, 1945; Lilienthal *et al.*, 1946; Pitts & Pace, 1947). Information on many of the categories listed is sketchy. Since carbon monoxide impairs oxygen transport, its effect is inevitably enhanced by any type of local or

Table 4.3: Factors Increasing Sensitivity to Carbon Monoxide
Accumulation

Category	Specific factors
Hypoxic conditions	Fetal life
	Anaemia
	Chronic obstructive lung disease
	Ischaemic heart disease
	Peripheral vascular disease
	Cerebral vascular disease
	High altitude residence
	Old age
Increased metabolism and/or respiratory minute volume	Physical work
	Pregnancy
	High altitude
	Thyrotoxicosis
	Newborn infants
	Hypoxic conditions
Increased endogenous production of carbon monoxide	Pregnancy
	Newborn child
	Haemolytic disease
	Saturation dives
Interaction with other drugs	Drug exposure (phenobarbital, diphenyl hydantoin, methylene chloride)
	Alcohol and depressant drugs
	Oxides of nitrogen
	Phenols and particulate matter

general oxygen lack (Bartlett, 1968; Dinman, 1968; Permutt & Farhi, 1969). Thus in patients with chronic chest disease an increase of the blood COHb from 1.43% to 4.08% decreased the time to severe exercise-induced shortness of breath from 219 to 147 seconds (Aronow *et al.*, 1977). An increase of oxygen demand (through such circumstances as physical work, pregnancy or thyrotoxicosis) also increases the chance that CO will induce tissue oxygen want (Smith *et al.*, 1935; Hellman & Pritchard, 1971). With short-term exposures, the associated increase of respiratory minute volume further augments the response relative to that seen during quiet resting ventilation (Cropp, 1970). The background body burden is further increased by exposure to polluted atmospheres in driving or at work, and through augmented endogenous production (a variety of situations where haemolysis is enhanced). In animal experiments, carbon monoxide enhances the effect of depressant drugs, including alcohol (Montgomery & Rubin, 1971; Pankow *et al.*, 1974); however, in man alcohol and CO apparently do not interact except at fairly high COHb levels — 12%

(Stewart *et al.*, 1974; Rockwell & Weir, 1975). Carbon monoxide may also add to the toxicity of other cigarette smoke constituents such as the oxides of nitrogen (Busey, 1972; Nakajima *et al.*, 1972) and phenol (Elfinova *et al.*, 1972).

All of the groups listed in Table 4.3 are more sensitive to CO-induced psychomotor disturbances than the general sedentary population, but in terms of the pathological problems that may arise, the patients with coronary and peripheral vascular disease are probably more vulnerable to CO than other categories, thus setting the permissible ceiling to CO accumulation.

Safe Level of Carbon Monoxide

The maximum acceptable concentration for the various constituents of tobacco smoke depends on the nature of the biological response. A substantial safety margin must be demanded for carcinogenesis, and (in the case of carbon monoxide exposure) an increase of vehicle accidents or cardiac fatalities. On the other hand, a minor disturbance of auditory vigilance that can be corrected by an increase of arousal or a small diminution in the speed for a one-mile run are of lesser concern.

A second consideration usually applied in studies of air pollutants is the universality of exposure. For example, a larger safety margin is needed to protect against general urban pollution with carbon monoxide than is required to counter the occasional accumulation of CO in a closed and poorly ventilated room. A third variable is the sensitivity of the test population. A wider margin must be allowed if the limit is based upon healthy young adults rather than a sensitive segment of the population (such as patients with ischaemic heart disease). Account must also be taken of half-life. Some of the toxic constituents of cigarette smoke remain in the body for a long period, but carbon monoxide is cleared with a half-time of three to four hours. Finally, there are questions of economics and practicality. Carbon monoxide can be brought down to quite modest levels if a smoky room is well-ventilated, but this imposes a high cost for heating and/or cooling; such expenditures may be difficult to justify if concentrations in the street outside a building are five to ten times higher than those inside!

The data presented in this chapter suggest that CO accumulation may have adverse effects upon psychomotor function and the course of ischaemic heart disease if the blood COHb exceeds 3%. Unfortunately, the baseline due to vehicle exhaust is a blood COHb of 1.0–1.5% in many large cities. It is thus not practicable to insist upon more than a twofold margin of safety. Even a 1.5% COHb reading may present some danger to a cardiac patient who is living at high altitude. A COHb of 1.5% is reached with exposure to 50 ppm of CO for 15 minutes, 15 ppm for one hour, or 9 ppm for eight hours; the latter two patterns of exposure are quite commonly encountered during passive smoking.

5 SMOKE EXPOSURE AND ACUTE CHANGES OF CARDIO-RESPIRATORY FUNCTION

Passive exposure to a dense cloud of tobacco smoke could induce acute changes of respiratory function through several mechanisms, including: (i) an emotional reaction to an unpleasant environment; (ii) mechanical stimulation of the airway by the particulate cloud; (iii) an irritant response to constituents of the gaseous or the particulate phase; (iv) a pharmacological reaction to nicotine; and (v) an allergic response to the tobacco itself, or to other smoke constituents. This chapter will review briefly the methodology of acute human exposure to cigarette smoke, the effects of such exposure upon cardiorespiratory function and the practical significance of data obtained from such experiments.

Test Methodology

Subjects

The subjects who volunteer for most passive exposure experiments are, not surprisingly, non-smokers. Often, they have a personal interest in respiratory problems which they believe to arise from the accumulation of tobacco smoke and this may bias responses — particularly the reporting of subjective reactions. Unfortunately, tobacco smoke is sufficiently obvious in terms of both its odour and the resultant haze that it is not possible to circumvent this difficulty through a 'double-blind' experimental design (where neither the subject nor the observer are aware of the days when exposure occurs). However, some attempt can be made to distinguish psychological from pharmacological reactions through the construction of a dose-response curve. Psychological reactions are likely to be precipitated by quite low doses and to show an erratic response to increases of smoke concentration; in contrast, a true pharmacological effect is likely to vary in a regular logarithmic or sigmoid fashion with exposure level.

Smokers and ex-smokers are also affected adversely by the environmental accumulation of tobacco smoke. However, there is some evidence that smokers show lesser pulmonary response to irritant gases than do non-smokers (Shephard *et al.*, in preparation), possible because a thick mucus film dilutes the irritant; they might thus tolerate passive smoking better than a non-smoker would. Questionnaire responses suggest that the ex-smoker also has some immunity to cigarette smoke

Table 5.1: Reported Influence of Passive Smoking Upon Health of 440 Non-smokers and 93 Ex-smokers

Effect	Non-smokers (%)	Ex-smokers (%)
None	11.6	37.6
Nuisance symptoms	46.8	37.6
Major effect on health	41.6	23.6

Source: Based on data from Shephard & LaBarre, 1976, 1978.

Table 5.2: Most Frequent Symptomatic Response to 'Passive Smoking' Reported by 440 Non-smokers and 93 Ex-smokers

	Percentage reporting symptom	
Symptom	Non-smoker	Ex-smoker
None	16.4	36.5
Headache	13.0	8.6
Stinging eyes	46.6	27.9
Running nose	2.5	1.0
Phlegm	0.7	1.0
Wheezing	2.7	2.1
Nausea	8.6	11.8
Dizziness	1.8	4.3
Other	7.7	6.4

Source: Based on data from Shephard *et al.*, 1978a.

(Table 5.1). One survey of Torontonians showed that only 11.6% of non-smokers were unaffected by passive exposure to cigarette smoke, while 41.6% thought it had a major effect upon their health; in contrast, 37.6% of ex-smokers were unaffected, and only 23.6% reported a major effect upon their health (Shephard & LaBarre, 1976, 1978). The most frequent complaint was stinging of the eyes (Table 5.2); possibly because of habituation from previous smoking, the ex-smokers were affected less frequently than the non-smokers. Visual complaints also became more frequent in older subjects, probably because sight was becoming more marginal (Shephard *et al.*, 1978a, b; 1979c).

Exposure Chamber

Exposure is conveniently carried out in a small booth (volume 14–15 m^3) with smooth walls and a minimum of furniture that could adsorb smoke. A window is required to allow continuous observation of the subject, and small ports in the wall are needed to pass cables to the recording apparatus. The smoke cloud is usually generated by a smoking machine (see Chapter 1); this has the advantage that the dose of pollutants can be controlled rather closely. Nevertheless, for greater realism a habitual smoker might be used to contaminate the chamber. A large airduct and evacuating fan in the ceiling is needed to clear the chamber air after each experiment.

Since most biological functions show a circadian rhythm, it is best to design experiments so that subjects perform both a true and a sham exposure at similar times on two randomly selected days. In our experience (Pimm *et al.*, 1978), realistic smoke concentrations are produced if the chamber is primed by the simultaneous smoking of four popular 85 mm filter cigarettes and concentrations of smoke are maintained by the burning of a further cigarette at 30-minute intervals. Smoke is lost through: (i) respiratory absorption by the subject and the technician; (ii) seepage around doors and through ceiling tiles; (iii) absorption in environmental monitoring devices; and (iv) natural clearance mechanisms (including coagulation, impaction, gravitational settling and various chemical reactions).

Figure 5.1: A Comparison Between the Theoretical and Actual Loss of Suspended Particulate Matter from a Small Chamber (Half-time 43 Minutes, Emission 17 mg per Cigarette, Chamber Volume 14.6 m^3)

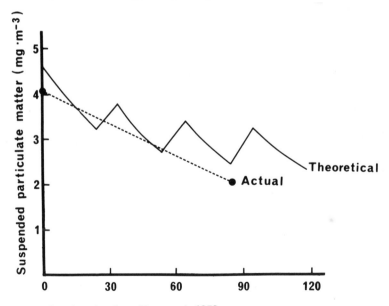

Source: Based on data from Pimm *et al.*, 1978.

Figure 5.2: A Comparison Between the Theoretical Loss of CO Due to Chemical Reactivity (Half-time of Reaction 84 Minutes, Further 85 ml Added every 30 Minutes) and Actual Loss from 14.6 m³ Chamber

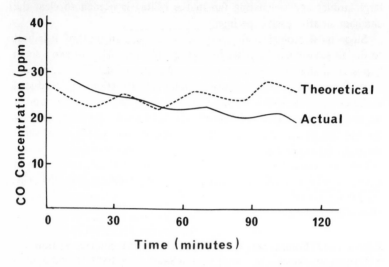

Source: Based on data from Pimm *et al.*, 1978.

Carbon monoxide concentrations are conveniently monitored by an electrochemical detector such as the 'Ecolyser'. Given a 14.6 m³ chamber volume, the smoking pattern adopted by Pimm *et al.* (1978) yielded an initial CO concentration of 28.5 ppm, some 24 ppm above ambient readings; this fell gradually to about 19.5 ppm over a two-hour exposure.

Suspended particulate matter can be determined by means of an electrostatic precipitator. In this device, a motor draws air samples into an electrically grounded cylindrical sampling tube. A high voltage is applied to a central electrode and an ionizing wire. The solid particles that are initially suspended in the air stream gain an electrical charge, and are repelled onto the cylinder wall. The cylinder is then removed and weighed. The particulate burden declines faster than carbon monoxide, due to growth, impaction and settling of the particles. In the experiments of Pimm *et al.* (1978) the concentration decreased from 4 mg·m⁻³ to 2 mg·m⁻³ over the first 90 minutes of observation. These findings agree fairly well with theoretical predictions based on a particulate emission of 17 mg per cigarette (Hoegg, 1972) and a half-life of 43 minutes for suspended particulate matter (Penkala & De Oliviera, 1975; Figure 5.1).

Carbon monoxide is a relatively stable component of the gas phase, although it apparently undergoes a slow chemical change when kept in a small room. It thus has a half-life of about 84 minutes (Penkala & De Oliviera, 1975). Given an emission of 85 ml of CO per cigarette (Hoegg, 1972), Pimm *et al.* (1978) found a somewhat more rapid disappearance of CO than could be explained by chemical reactivity alone (Figure 5.2); they attributed this to the other routes of loss discussed above.

Some chemical constituents undergo a more rapid change than carbon monoxide, which complicates the interpretation of results. Nevertheless, the chamber atmosphere is realistic of 'real-life' conditions in that 'passive-smoking' normally involves the breathing of a mixture of recent and aged smoke.

Effects Upon Cardio-respiratory Function

Cardiovascular System

It is well recognized that smoking increases the heart rate of the smoker, both at rest (Thomas *et al.*, 1956; Regan *et al.*, 1961; Irving & Yamomoto, 1963; Herxheimer *et al.*, 1967; Armitage *et al.*, 1975, 1978) and in exercise (Blackburn *et al.*, 1960; Chevalier *et al.*, 1963). There is an associated increase of both cardiac output and systemic blood pressure (Behr *et al.*, 1981). There may also be a decrease in end-systolic volume and in pulmonary transit time (Behr *et al.*, 1981). Comroe (1964) attributed these various changes to the action of nicotine upon the chemosensitive tissue in the carotid bodies, although the more usually accepted explanation is that the nicotine induces a release of the hormone noradrenaline (Burn, 1960; Cryer *et al.*, 1976). Blood flow to the skin is diminished (Shepherd, 1951), flow to the muscles is increased (Rottenstein *et al.*, 1960) and the irritability of the heart muscle is augmented with an enhanced liability to abnormalities of heart rhythm (Emele, 1975). All of these changes disappear over the first six hours of abstinence from cigarettes (Rode *et al.*, 1972).

The evidence that similar changes occur during passive smoking is not particularly strong. Luquette *et al.* (1970) exposed 40 ten-year-old children to a smoke-filled atmosphere in groups of three. The students showed an insignificant increase of heart rate, and a significant increase of systolic blood pressure relative to control days, but these changes could have been induced by overall excitement, since films on the harmful effects of smoking were shown during exposure. Harke & Bleichert (1972) found no changes of heart rate, blood pressure,

Figure 5.3: The Influence of Chamber Exposure to Cigarette Smoke Upon the Resting Heart Rate

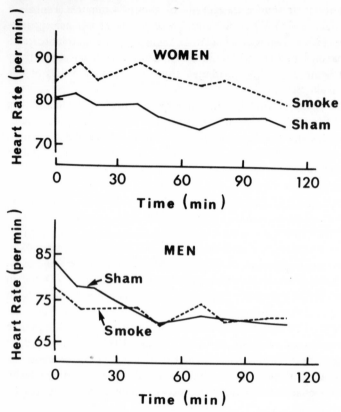

Source: Based on data from Pimm *et al.*, 1978.

electrocardiogram or skin blood flow despite severe exposure conditions. Rummel *et al.* (1975) attempted to distinguish physiological and psychological reactions to cigarette smoke. They divided a sample of 56 students into those who were indifferent and those who actively disliked exposure. Both groups showed an increase of systolic blood pressure during the experiment, but the latter group had a higher heart rate throughout. Pimm *et al.* (1978) observed a 5-10 beat per minute increase of resting heart rate in women throughout exposure; however, it is hard to attribute this to a pharmacological response, since male subjects showed no increase of resting heart rate under the same conditions (Figure 5.3). The exercise heart rates of the female subjects were also increased during the first few minutes of exposure days, but again the absence of a parallel increase in the men suggests this was a psychological rather than a pharmacological response to the smoke cloud.

Aronow (1978) described a 38% shortening of the time to angina, when volunteers with ischaemic heart disease exercised in an unventilated room that was occupied by smokers. Although the patients showed some increase of blood carboxyhaemoglobin level in these experiments, the end-point (the reported onset of anginal pain) is necessarily subjective. It is difficult to imagine that enclosure in a very smoky room did not have some emotional impact upon patients who were liable to angina, and the psychological disturbance may have done more to hasten the onset of symptoms than the increase of blood carboxyhaemoglobin.

Data on nicotine absorption during passive smoking have been discussed already (see Chapter 3). Even under very adverse conditions, the urinary nicotine excretion of a non-smoker is only a small fraction (6-7%) of that seen in a smoker (Russell & Feyerabend, 1975). In effect, the non-smoker eliminates nicotine almost as fast as it is absorbed, and in such circumstances it is unlikely that a sufficient quantity of the drug will accumulate to exert a pharmacological effect.

Respiratory System

The acute effects of cigarette smoke upon the respiratory tract include: (i) a depression of function in the ciliae lining the airway; (ii) a stimulation of mucus production by the goblet cells of the bronchial lining; and (iii) a varying amount of bronchospasm. Chronic exposure may cause chronic bronchitis, emphysema and various forms of lung cancer.

The immediate reaction of the ciliae may be a transient stimulation of activity, but if the exposure continues, their rate of movement is depressed for as long as 30 to 40 minutes (Dalhamn, 1966; Camner *et al.*, 1973; Thomson & Pavia, 1973; Wanner *et al.*, 1973). Ciliary depression has been attributed to a variety of toxic constituents in the smoke, including hydrogen cyanide, acrolein and certain of the aldehydes. The importance of ciliary inhibition is that it impairs a vital mechanism for the removal of mucus toxic particulate matter, viruses and bacteria from the airways. For this reason, passive smoking could increase the chances of developing acute respiratory infections, adverse reactions to industrial dusts such as asbestos and uranium and chronic bronchitis (Shephard, 1978b). However, it must be stressed that a number of the experiments showing ciliary toxicity have been conducted on animals where the cigarette smoke was admitted directly to the trachea via a tracheostomy tube. Under more normal circumstances, when air is inhaled via the nose − or even the mouth − some of the toxic constituents may be removed from the airstream before the ciliae are reached. Yeates *et al.* (1975) observed a slowing of clearance in man, but Camner *et al.* (1971) found an acceleration even with vigorous smoking.

The increased production of bronchial mucus (Reid, 1960; Ebert & Terracio, 1975) has little acute effect − it may even offer some protection against irritant gases (Shephard *et al.*, in preparation). However, over a longer period, accumulation of mucus brings about the typical picture of chronic bronchitis, with poor mixing of inspired gas and airway obstruction (Mertens *et al.*, 1978; Shephard, 1976).

Spasm of the airways (Nadel & Comroe, 1961; Clarke *et al.*, 1970; DaSilva & Hamosh, 1973; Hamosh & DaSilva, 1977) varies with the size of the inhaled particles (Covert & Frank, 1980), the route of inhalation (nasal or oral) and the sensitivity of the individual's bronchial tree (Gayrard *et al.*, 1974). The typical response of a smoker to a single cigarette is an immediate doubling of airway resistance, with a gradual return to normal over the next 30–40 minutes. However, in an older subject with some chronic bronchitis the rate of recovery may be slower. One practical consequence is a proportionate increase in the oxygen cost of breathing (Rode & Shephard, 1971). While this has little significance under resting conditions, it can seriously restrict maximum effort. The bronchospasm does not seem to be a pharmacological response to nicotine, since similar changes are seen with normal and low nicotine content cigarettes (Comroe, 1964; Reintjes *et al.*, 1972). The reaction is enhanced by beta adrenergic blocking drugs such as propranolol (Zuskin *et al.*, 1974), but is reversed by atropine (Sterling, 1967). It thus seems that a vagal reflex is involved. The stimulus may be the dense cloud of particles itself, as in some industrial situations (Dautrebande & DuBois, 1958; McDermott, 1962); it may be a reaction to CO_2 (unlikely, since this gas usually causes bronchodilatation); or it may be a reaction to irritant components in the vapour phase of the smoke (Guillerm *et al.*, 1972). Aviado *et al.* (1966) have suggested histamine release is involved. If irritants are responsible, it is worth stressing that their concentration is greater in sidestream than in mainstream smoke.

Because the tobacco particles are so small (see Chapter 1), they penetrate readily to the finer branches of the airway, and the main site of spasm is probably the small, muscular bronchioles. Unfortunately, these finer air passages contribute relatively little to the overall airway resistance, and the disturbance of function may be greater than indicated by simple respiratory function tests (which examine mainly large airway resistance). In theory, the optimum tools for demonstration of a response to cigarette smoke are specific measures of small airway function such as the frequency dependence of lung compliance, the critical closing volume, flow-volume curves and the modification of respiratory airflow by the use of helium/oxygen mixtures (Dosman *et al.*, 1975; Martin *et al.*, 1975; Cherniack, 1977; Knudson *et al.*, 1977; Oxhøj *et al.*, 1977). Gas distribution is impaired by the small airway narrowing, and this decreases the effectiveness of ventilation in terms of gas exchange (Wilson *et al.*, 1960; Ross *et al.*, 1967).

The author's laboratory has conducted sequences of lung function tests under conditions where non-smokers have undergone two-hour chamber exposures to cigarette smoke. In the first series of experiments, subjects sat at rest in a room of 14.6 m^3 (Pimm *et al.*, 1978). The main complaints were of eye irritation and nasal discharge, and the only common respiratory symptom was coughing. There was apparently a sex difference of response. In men, residual volume and functional residual capacity increased significantly relative to control days, but in women there was no such change (Table 5.3). This result could possibly arise through a combination of small airway spasm and sympathetic activation. In the men, it could be argued that spasm predominated, with resultant changes of static lung volumes, but in the women sympathetic activation was sufficient to reverse any tendency to airway narrowing. The increase of heart rate, seen in women but not in men, would support such a view, as would measurements of maximum expiratory flow at 25% of vital capacity (Table 5.4, some restriction in the men, but not in the women).

In a second experiment (Shephard *et al.*, 1979a), it was decided to test more adverse conditions. The initial 'loading' of the chamber was in some instances increased by the simultaneous burning of six cigarettes (CO concentration 31 ppm), while all subjects were required to perform intermittent exercise sufficient to increase the respiratory minute volume by a factor of 2.5. Grading the severity of symptoms, 12 subjects exposed to the initial loading of four cigarettes each accumulated an average of 10.3 symptom points, while ten subjects exposed to the six cigarette loading each accumulated an average of 13.8 sympton points (Table 5.5). The main symptoms were of odour and eye irritation, and only one of 23 volunteers reported wheezing and tightness in the chest. He did not show any unusual impairment of his flow/

Table 5.3: Changes of Static Lung Volumes Observed with Two-hour Passive Exposure to Cigarette Smoke

Variable	Sham exposure		Test exposure	
	0 min	120 min	0 min	120 min
Vital capacity (l)				
Men	5.74	5.70	5.75	5.71
Women	3.48	3.60	3.54	3.53
Functional residual capacity (l)				
Men	3.39	3.37	3.38	3.53[a]
Women	2.26	2.23	2.22	2.20
Residual volume (l)				
Men	1.40	1.34	1.38	1.49[a]
Women	1.02	0.98	0.99	1.02
Total lung capacity (l)				
Men	7.14	7.04	7.13	7.20
Women	4.50	4.58	4.54	4.55

Note: a. $P < 0.05$.
Source: Based on data for healthy men and women from Pimm *et al.*, 1978.

Table 5.4: Changes of Dynamic Lung Volumes over Two-hour Passive Exposure to Cigarette Smoke

Variable	Sham exposure		Test exposure	
	0 min	120 min	0 min	120 min
Forced vital capacity (l)				
Men	5.36	5.41	5.38	5.46
Women	3.41	3.46	3.45	3.49
One second forced exp. vol. (l)				
Men	4.35	4.50	4.36	4.53
Women	2.94	3.06	3.03	3.07
Max. exp. flow at 50% of vital capacity ($l \cdot sec^{-1}$)				
Men	5.04	5.32	5.04	5.26
Women	4.21	4.25	4.10	4.23
Max. exp. flow at 25% of vital capacity ($l \cdot sec^{-1}$)				
Men	2.25	2.53	2.38	2.45[a]
Women	2.07	2.08	2.01	2.09

Note: a. Lesser increase of $\dot{V}_{max}$ (25% vc) at 90 minutes of test exposure ($P < 0.05$).
Source: Based on flow/volume data for healthy men and women from Pimm *et al.*, 1978.

Table 5.5: Symptoms Reported by Subjects Performing Intermittent Exercise While Exposed to Either 4 + 3 or 6 + 3 Cigarettes in a 14.6 m³ Chamber

Symptom	Average symptom score[a]	
	4 + 3 cigarettes	6 + 3 cigarettes
Odour	2.9	4.0
Nausea	0	0.3
Cough	0	0.9
Sputum	0.1	0.0
Sore throat	0.6[b]	0.6[b]
Shortness of breath	0.3	0.4
Nasal discharge or stuffiness	0.6	1.3
Wheezing	0	0.1
Tightness in chest	0	0.2
Dizziness	0.4	0.7
Fatigue	0.3	0.4[b]
Eye irritation	3.3	3.8
Headache	0.6	0.9
Other	0	0
Total	10.3	13.8

Notes: a. 1 = trace; 5 = very severe.
    b. Also reported in one sham exposure.
Source: Based on data from Shephard *et al.*, 1979.

volume curve. The respiratory minute volume was increased 10–20% during exposure of the intermittent exercisers to the cigarette smoke, but there was no evidence of any increase in functional residual or residual gas volumes; indeed, there was a slight and statistically insignificant trend to a decrease of expiratory reserve and functional residual capacity (Table 5.6). On the other hand, the dynamic lung volumes all tended to be depressed relative to sham exposure days (Table 5.7). Furthermore, there was little evidence of any adaptation over the two-hour exposure — indeed, the final results showed slightly greater functional losses than those observed in the first few minutes of the experiment.

The general conclusion from these experiments is that the acute effects of realistic cigarette smoke concentrations upon the respiratory tract are quite limited. There are several possible explanations for this. First, the dose of both particulate matter and irritant aldehydes is small relative to that encountered during active smoking. The calculation of 'cigarette equivalents' is hazardous, but nevertheless the average sedentary subject is unlikely to respire more than 1 m³ of air over a two-hour

Table 5.6: Changes of Static Lung Volumes Observed with Two-hour Passive Cigarette Smoke Exposure

Variable	Sham exposure (% pre-exposure control)	Experimental exposure (% pre-exposure control)
Vital capacity		
4 + 3 cigs.	102.7 ± 6.9	101.2 ± 3.9
6 + 3 cigs.	102.9 ± 4.8	103.2 ± 2.3
Functional residual capacity		
4 + 3 cigs.	101.0 ± 14.3	96.7 ± 12.7
6 + 3 cigs.	104.7 ± 14.3	98.2 ± 8.1
Residual volume		
4 + 3 cigs.	98.7 ± 27.9	102.2 ± 32.9
6 + 3 cigs.	109.3 ± 20.0	100.5 ± 15.6
Total lung capacity		
4 + 3 cigs.	99.9 ± 10.1	99.9 ± 6.9
6 + 3 cigs.	104.1 ± 3.3	103.0 ± 2.0

Source: Based on data for healthy exercising adults from Shephard *et al.*, 1979.

Table 5.7: Changes of Dynamic Lung Volumes Observed over Two-hour Passive Cigarette Smoke Exposure

Variable	Sham exposure (% pre-exposure control)	Experimental exposure (% pre-exposure control)
Forced vital capacity		
4 + 3 cigs.	99.7 ± 9.3	92.3 ± 4.1
6 + 3 cigs.	100.9 ± 4.9	99.4 ± 8.1
One second forced exp. vol.		
4 + 3 cigs.	103.3 ± 7.0	101.1 ± 9.1
6 + 3 cigs.	101.1 ± 7.7	99.9 ± 7.0
Max. exp. flow at 50% VC		
4 + 3 cigs.	110.2 ± 19.6	102.7 ± 15.0
6 + 3 cigs.	102.9 ± 10.9	102.7 ± 15.9
Max. exp. flow at 25% VC		
4 + 3 cigs.	113.1 ± 26.9	106.4 ± 20.1
6 + 3 cigs.	112.1 ± 19.6	105.1 ± 27.1

Source: Based on data for healthy exercising adults from Shephard *et al.*, 1979.

exposure. The particulate cloud inhaled thus weighs about 3 mg, compared with the emission of 17 mg or more from a single cigarette; at worst, the passive exposure is equivalent to about 0.2 of a cigarette, spaced over two hours. Secondly, the active smoker inhales via the mouth, whereas the passive smoker usually breathes through the nose in both rest and light exercise (nasal inspiration continues up to a ventilation of 35 $1 \cdot min^{-1}$, Niinimaa *et al.*, 1979); thus, a portion of the particulate matter may be filtered from the airstream in the nose. Thirdly, the primary response of bronchospasm is readily reversed by adrenergic activity, so that fear or annoyance caused by the smoke exposure could counteract a direct action of particulate matter upon receptors in the airways. Finally, it is well-recognized that the spasm induced by cigarette smoke undergoes a transient and partial reversal during the deep inspiration needed for recording of a flow-volume loop. These various factors may explain why only minor changes of static and dynamic lung volumes have been observed during and following exposure to the cigarette smoke.

Exercise Response

The exercise response gives some indication of the overall impact of cigarette smoke upon the cardio-respiratory system. Any increase of blood carboxyhaemoglobin decreases exercise tolerance (see Chapter 4). Vigorous exercise in itself stimulates the secretion of catecholamines and, perhaps for this reason, the acute sympatho-mimetic effects of smoking are less apparent during physical activity than under resting conditions. The heart rate averages about five beats per minute faster in the smoker than in the non-smoker at a given intensity of sub-maximal work (Blackburn *et al.*, 1960; Chevalier *et al.*, 1963; Rode *et al.*, 1972), although the maximum heart rate is the same in smokers and non-smokers. There have been suggestions that the oxygen debt is larger in smokers (Chevalier *et al.*, 1963), but this does not seem an acute pharmacological response, since the situation is not corrected by a period of abstinence from cigarettes (Henry & Fitzhenry, 1950). Possibly, it reflects a chronic effect upon the blood flow to the calf muscles.

Animal experiments have demonstrated a decrease of treadmill endurance time (Hrubes & Baettig, 1970), with an increase of post-exercise blood lactate, glutamic oxaloacetic transaminase and creatine phosphokinase concentrations (Reece & Ball, 1972) following acute passive exposure to cigarette smoke. In human experiments from our laboratory (Pimm *et al.*, 1978; Shephard *et al.*, 1979a), healthy adults

Table 5.8: Exercise Response of Subjects Immediately Following Two-hour Passive Exposure to Cigarette Smoke

Variable	Men		Women	
	Sham exposure	Experimental exposure	Sham exposure	Experimental exposure
Respiratory minute volume ($l \cdot min^{-1}$)	75.3	77.9[a]	48.1	48.3
Respiratory rate (breaths per min)	28.3	29.3	31.5	30.7
Tidal volume (ml)	2,661	2,659	1,527	1,573
Heart rate (beats per min)	158	160	164	169[a]
Oxygen consumption ($l \cdot min^{-1}$)	2.47	2.65[b]	1.51	1.48

Notes: Differences between sham and experimental exposure:
    a. $P < 0.01$.
    b. $P < 0.05$.
Source: Based on data from Pimm *et al.*, 1978.

Table 5.9: Responses to Sub-maximal Exercise During Passive Cigarette Smoke Exposure (Average of Data for Minutes 54, 84 and 114 of Two-hour Exposure, Expressed as Per Cent of Pre-exposure Resting Values)

Variable	4 + 3 cigarettes		6 + 3 cigarettes	
	Sham exposure (%)	Experimental exposure (%)	Sham exposure (%)	Experimental exposure (%)
Respiratory minute volume	242	265	214	238
Respiratory rate	128	126	162	152
Tidal volume	189	210	132	157

Source: Based on data from Shephard *et al.*, 1979a.

showed a modest smoke-induced increase of respiratory minute volumes during and after exercise when data were compared between sham and experimental exposures (Tables 5.8 and 5.9). The increase of ventilation in most instances reflected an increase of tidal volume rather than respiratory rate (Tables 5.8 and 5.9). There was also a suggestion of an increase in the oxygen cost of work in men but not in women; this was probably a combined effect of an increase of ventilation (Shephard, 1966) and some increase in the oxygen cost of unit ventilation (Rode & Shephard, 1971).

None of the changes in exercise performance were of sufficient magnitude to be of practical importance, except for the athlete competing in an event demanding an outstanding oxygen transport capacity.

Practical Significance

Basis of Observed Responses

While the cardio-respiratory changes observed in the active smoker are determined by local reactions to particulate matter and irritant vapours, plus systemic reactions to nicotine, it is less clear that the minor reactions described during passive exposure of the non-smoker have a similar basis. Certainly, the respired doses of particulate matter and of nicotine are insufficient to provoke a true pharmacological response. On the other hand, there are relatively high concentrations of various irritants in sidestream smoke (Chapter 2, Table 2.1), and the industrial threshold limit for several noxious chemicals is surpassed when smoke accumulates in small, poorly ventilated rooms (Table 3.4). There is little question that concentrations are sufficient to stimulate conjunctival receptors, and a similar irritant reaction might be postulated in the respiratory tract. However, detailed inspection of the respiratory data does not suggest this is a particularly plausible explanation. Stimulation of tracheal irritant receptors tends to curtail inspiratory drive, with a decrease of tidal volume and a compensatory increase of respiratory rate (Folinsbee *et al.*, 1975). In contrast, the trend in the passive smoking experiments is to an increase of tidal volume. This could conceivably be attributed to a greater peripheral drive (for example, an action of absorbed nicotine upon the carotid chemoreceptors) but, as already stressed, the passive absorption of nicotine is insufficient to exert such an effect. The onset of hyperventilation before exposure, with a decreasing discrepancy between sham and experimental days as the experiment continues and the absence of a clear dose/response curve, support an alternative hypothesis (central facilitation of respiratory drive due to an emotional reaction to the smoke exposure). The slight tachycardia seems in keeping with this latter explanation.

Implications for an Air Quality Criterion

It could be argued that if passive exposure to cigarette smoke was causing a clear physiological or pharmacological response of the cardio-respiratory system, then the level of smoke in the environment was unacceptably high. However, the experimental data provide only meagre and somewhat inconsistent evidence that the respiratory tract of healthy subjects reacts to cigarette smoke, either at rest or with the added stress of moderate exercise. It thus seems likely that the air quality criterion will be determined by other considerations such as subjective tolerance, impairment of vision, chronic health effects and the responses of sensitive populations such as those with asthma or angina.

6 ACUTE EFFECTS OF CIGARETTE SMOKE UPON OTHER BODY SYSTEMS

This chapter will look briefly at other ways in which passive exposure to cigarette smoke affects the body — particularly its effects upon the eyes and nose, with resultant annoyance and physical symptoms.

Effects upon the Eyes

Active Smoking

Adverse ophthalmic effects of active smoking include glaucoma (Bahna & Bjerkedal, 1975; Morgan & Drance, 1975; Mehra et al., 1976; Shephard et al., 1978b), cyanide-induced optic neuritis (Foulds et al., 1969; Crews et al., 1970; Rossman, 1970; Chisholm et al., 1971; Wilson et al., 1971; Chisholm, 1972; Jayle et al., 1972; Bhargava, 1973; Pettigrew & Fell, 1973; Potts, 1973; Durazzini et al., 1975; Perdriel et al., 1975; Perkin et al., 1975; Perkin & Rose, 1976), corneal arcus (Rosenmann et al., 1974) and vascular changes in the retina (Parke, 1975; Perdriel, 1975).

The majority of these changes develop over many years of heavy tobacco usage, and are unlikely to result from the lesser smoke concentrations encountered by the non-smoker during normal daily life. However, the eyes are quite sensitive to nicotine. A nicotine-induced spasm of the retinal blood vessels can change the visual acuity of some subjects from 20/20 to 20/60 in as little as five minutes (Parke, 1975), the required stimulus being provided by the smoking of as little as one cigarette. Again, a rise of intraocular pressure of 5 mm Hg has been reported in 11.4% of normal subjects and 37.1% of primary glaucoma patients within five minutes of smoking a single cigarette (Mehra et al., 1976). The chain of events postulated by Mehra et al. (1976) was a nicotine-induced intraocular vasoconstriction, a rise of episcleral venous pressure and a restriction of the normal outflow of aqueous humour from the angle of the eye, although other authors have queried whether smoking does indeed influence the formation or the outflow of aqueous humour (Bahna & Bjerkedal, 1975).

Certain effects of carbon monoxide upon visual vigilance, depth perception, visual field and glare recovery have been discussed in Chapter 4. Ophthalmologists have attributed some of the acute smoking-induced disturbances of visual physiology to nicotine rather than carbon monoxide absorption (Krippner & Heimstra, 1969; Conraux & Collard, 1975); such problems include a restriction of the visual field (particularly when the intensity of illumination is low; Scoughton & Heimstra, 1973), impaired reactions to dazzling light (Buratowski *et al.*, 1974), a change in the rapid phase of nystagmus (Conraux & Collard, 1975), and a depression of the electro-oculogram (Schmidt, 1970; Francois *et al.*, 1974; but not Haase & Muller, 1971).

Subjective Reactions in Passive Smoking

In confirmation of previous studies (Johansson & Ronge, 1965; Speer, 1971; Portheine, 1972; Anderson & Dalhamn, 1973; Johansson, 1976; Weber *et al.*, 1976b; Weber-Tschoop *et al.*, 1976a) and our studies upon break-up of the human tear film (Basu *et al.*, 1978), eye irritation seems the main complaint during passive exposure to cigarette smoke (Table 5.5). Speer (1971) questioned non-allergic subjects concerning their reactions to cigarette smoke; 69% complained of eye irritation, 32% of headache, 29% of nasal symptoms and 25% of cough. Johansson & Ronge (1965, 1966) noted that cigarette smoke produced the greatest amount of irritation when the air was warm and dry; a small increase of ambient humidity was often sufficient to relieve the situation. Johansson (1976) further commented that while smokers were prone to eye irritation, nasal irritation was also a common complaint of non-smokers. Shephard *et al.* (1978a, 1979c) observed that elderly non-smokers were more frequently bothered by cigarettes than by smoke from other types of fire, but in young people the reverse was true (Table 6.1).

Johansson & Ronge (1965, 1966) set the threshold concentration at which a cigarette smoke cloud was reported as 'unpleasant' at an average of 4.7 $mg \cdot m^{-3}$ particulates for a non-smoker, and 9 $mg \cdot m^{-3}$ for a smoker. However, the eye irritation threshold (9 $mg \cdot m^{-3}$) was similar for smokers and non-smokers. This last figure is surprisingly high. Anderson & Dalhamn (1973) and Pimm *et al.* (1978) both found that most non-smokers were reporting eye irritation at particulate levels of 2–4 $mg \cdot m^{-3}$.

On public service vehicles, one possible remedy is some segregation of smokers and non-smokers. The US Federal Aviation Administration (1971) questioned aircraft passengers, and found that 84% of those complaining about smoke accumulation would be content with a segregation arrangement. Seiff (1973) noted that four out of six subjects developed eye irritation when smoking on a bus was unrestricted (CO concentration 33 ppm), but that when smoking was restricted to the

Table 6.1: Percentage of Subjects Noting Lachrymation with Passive Exposure to Cigarette Smoke, Active Smoking and Exposure to Other Types of Smoke

Group	Passive smoking		Active smoking		Other types of smoke	
	Men %	Women %	Men %	Women %	Men %	Women %
Non-smokers	60.0	52.2	—	—	54.3	66.2
Ex-smokers	78.3	62.0	23.7	8.0	39.1	34.0
Smokers	36.1	40.2	23.0	19.5	45.9	37.9

Source: Based on data from Shephard *et al.*, 1979c.

Table 6.2: Annoyance of Non-smokers by a Cigarette Smouldering in an Ashtray and by Active Smoking

Source of smoke	Per cent of subjects annoyed	
	Men (%)	Women (%)
Smouldering cigarette	45.7	41.9
Active smoking	23.9	28.7

Source: Based on data from Shephard *et al.*, 1979c.

rear 20% of seats (CO concentration 18 ppm) none of the six developed eye irritation.

Inside buildings, the accumulation of smoke depends upon the efficiency of ventilation. Johansson & Ronge (1966) concluded that a ventilation rate of 12 m³ per hour per cigarette was necessary to avoid eye irritation, and that this had to be increased to 50 m³ per hour per cigarette in order to prevent the accumulation of unpleasant tobacco odours. A subsequent report from Johansson (1976) noted a difference of sensitivity between smokers and non-smokers; smokers were satisfied with a ventilation of 15 m³/h/cigarette, but non-smokers demanded a ventilation of 30 m³/h/cigarette to avoid eye irritation, and 60 m³/h/cigarette to avoid the odour of cigarette smoke. Weber *et al.* (1976b) based their ventilation standard upon the total number of cigarettes smoked. In a room of 30 m³, the burning of five cigarettes induced subjective complaints from 50% of occupants, while ten cigarettes produced strong or very strong eye irritation in 9% of subjects. Unlike Johansson & Ronge (1965) or Shephard *et al.* (1978a, b), Weber *et al.* (1976b) found somewhat greater eye irritation in smokers than in non-smokers.

As might be predicted from the respective irritant contents of mainstream and sidestream smoke (Table 2.1), more annoyance is caused by smouldering cigarettes than by active smoking (Table 6.2). Weber-Tschoop *et al.* (1976) separated the gas phase from total sidestream smoke, and concluded that while the gas phase was largely responsible for annoyance, irritation was arising mainly from the particulate phase.

Lachrymation

Both ex-smokers and continuing smokers seem more likely to lachrymate with passive than with active smoking (Shephard *et al.*, 1978a, 1979c), and they also react more to cigarettes than to other types of smoke (Table 6.1). More than half of non-smokers and ex-smokers and almost 40% of smokers report some lachrymation with passive exposure to cigarette smoke. However, it is generally reported as 'a little' rather than 'moderate' or 'heavy', and for this reason many subjects find it difficult to pinpoint the time to onset of this phenomenon. Some respond immediately, but complaints are most common after 5–15 minutes of exposure in female non-smokers, 20–30 minutes in male non-smokers and more than 60 minutes in ex-smokers and continuing smokers of both sexes. Heavy smokers, in particular, are late in noticing the symptom. Weber *et al.* (1976b) have noted similar timing to that reported by Shephard *et al.* (1978a, 1979c). In the German study, there was little response in less than five minutes, 50% response at ten minutes and fully developed symptoms at 20 minutes. Weber *et al.* (1976b) commented that the various manifestations of eye irritation (itching, tear-flow, eye-closing and eye-rubbing) developed roughly in parallel. Subjective eye irritation was strongly correlated with eye-blinking rate. The smoking of ten cigarettes in a 30 m^3 room doubled the blinking rate in 78% of subjects, and 70% of subjects 'wished to leave the room'. Experimental exposures to pure acrolein (0.3 ppm) caused eye irritation after 10–20 minutes (Weber-Tschoop *et al.*, 1977b); however, the response was usually much less than with cigarette smoke, suggesting that the effects of the smoke were due to a variety of irritant chemicals. Similar studies with formaldehyde showed irritation at a concentration of 1–2 ppm; again, the pure formaldehyde was considered less annoying than cigarette smoke (Weber-Tschoop *et al.*, 1977a). Glasson & Heuss (1977) ranked a number of chemicals in terms of their irritancy to the eyes, and concluded that formaldehyde and peroxy-acetylnitrite were the most irritant of the compounds evaluated.

The substantial delay in lachrymation presumably reflects time required for: (i) the build-up of a threshold concentration of irritant; and (ii) the penetration of the conjunctiva. Much depends upon the atmospheric concentration of the irritant and on the thickness of the initial tear film. The author (unpublished data) once had the experience of testing known concentrations of a pure irritant solution (malononitrile) on the conjunctiva of volunteer subjects. Typically, it took 3–4 minutes for an effective dose of irritant to penetrate to the receptor endings, causing pain; however, the response became more rapid as the concentration of the solution was increased. For reasons of safety, the irritant solutions were instilled into the periphery of the eyes, and it seems likely that a faster reaction would have been obtained if solutions had been dropped over the central part of the eyes (as occurs during passive smoking).

Tear Film, Lachrymation and Irritation

Stinging of the eyes seems a less common response to cigarette smoke than lachrymation. Shephard *et al.* (1978a, 1979c) found that the severity of irritation was inversely correlated with the severity of lachrymation (for non-smokers, $r = -0.52$; for ex-smokers, $r = -0.40$). The younger subjects tended to develop stinging of the eyes, while the older subjects lachrymated.

Basu *et al.* (1978) examined the possible contribution of changes in tear film composition to the process of eye irritation. The pre-corneal tear film of the normal eye is a continuous, stable layer, about 6 μm thick, which covers the exposed portions of the eye (Figure 6.1). Between blinking of the eyes, the integrity of the film is maintained by: (i) the mucus secretion of conjunctival goblet cells (the mucus content facilitates the spreading of the tear film over the corneal epithelium); and (ii) an outer lipid film secreted by the Meibomian glands (the lipid layer reduces evaporation from the water phase of the tear film; Wilson *et al.*, 1975). Deterioration in the stability of the tear film may impair the optical properties of the corneal surface (Grayson & Keates, 1969) and it also increases the risk of conjunctival infection (Dohlman *et al.*, 1976). The characteristics of the tear film are readily examined with a slit-lamp if the conjunctiva has been touched lightly with a fluorescein paper strip (Lemp & Hamill, 1973). After ten minutes of passive exposure to cigarette smoke (CO concentration about 24 ppm), the time to breakup of the tear film is shortened from a normal value of 25–30 seconds to about 13 seconds (Basu *et al.*, 1978). Several explanations may be advanced for this observation. Possibly, irritation increases blinking and rubbing of the eyes, with the mechanical stimulation

Figure 6.1: Structure of the Pre-corneal Tear Film

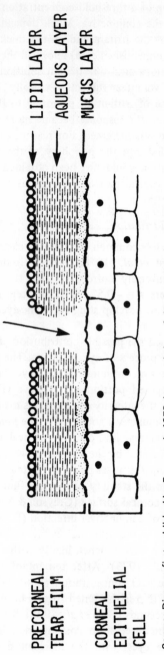

Source: Diagram first published by Basu et al., 1978; by permission of the Canadian Journal of Ophthalmology.

influencing the volume and chemical composition of the tears; however, the observations were made close to the onset of symptoms, and it is thus unlikely that rubbing of the eyes was a major factor altering tear composition. It is conceivable that aldehydes and oxidants in tobacco smoke could cause peroxidation of the lipid film, but again it is unlikely that such changes would be far advanced after only ten minutes of exposure. A more promising hypothesis is that the irritant components of the smoke alter the relative proportions of the three tear-film constituents. Basu *et al.* (1971) showed that acrolein 2-propenal caused an oculo-cardiac reflex in animals, and Waheed & Basu (1970) also reported an action of polluted air upon the conjunctival goblet cells. Lemp *et al.* (1971) noted that although the breakup time varied when the tear film was deficient in aqueous constituents, it was always low in eyes where mucus secretion was impaired. Certainly, the experiments of Basu *et al.* (1978) suggest some action upon tear-film secretion, but further observations are needed to resolve whether there is simply a local or reflex stimulation of watery secretion, or whether there is also a reduced secretion of the stabilizing constituents of the tear film.

Effects on Vision

A small percentage (13.5%) of the subjects surveyed by Shephard *et al.* (1978a) believed that on occasion passive exposure to cigarette smoke affected their vision. This response was made less often by the older subjects — our data support the hypothesis that irritation led to conjunctival suffusion (as during hay fever), and that such a response was less likely if the irritant material was diluted and/or washed away by lachrymation. About one-third of those reporting a visual problem noted immediate recovery on leaving the smoke-filled room. This would be unlikely if there had been severe conjunctival suffusion. However, almost a third of those affected reported that symptoms persisted for 15 or more minutes after exposure. The effect on vision was no more frequent in subjects who wore glasses for reading; possibly, the lenses offered some protection against irritant particles.

Effects Upon the Nose

Active Smoking

The nose is somewhat immune to the adverse effects of active smoking, since most smokers inhale and exhale smoke via the mouth. Nevertheless, a proportion of subjects allow some smoke to escape via the nose; this is particularly likely to occur in an individual who chooses to inhale rather than trapping the smoke in his or her mouth. According to Kittel (1976), heavy smoking causes chronic inflammatory swelling of the nasal mucosa, while pyridines and colloidins in the smoke damage the receptor cells, impairing the sense of smell (Arfmann & Chapanis, 1962; Joyner, 1964; Matzker, 1965). There is also some increase in the risk of nasal carcinoma in heavy smokers (Calvet & Coll, 1968; Farago, 1968).

Passive Smoking

In contrast, the nose of the non-smoker is relatively vulnerable, since a person who is passively exposed to cigarette smoke breathes through the nose unless required to speak, sing or perform vigorous exercise. The nose filters out up to 90% of soluble gases (Oberst, 1961) and a substantial fraction of the particulate matter (Dorman, 1971). Symptoms may reflect reactions to acrolein and similar irritants (Feron *et al.*, 1978), pharmacological effects of nicotine on the vasculature of the nose, allergic reactions and psychologically-induced alterations in nasal calibre.

Complaints include odour, nasal discharge and nasal obstruction (Pimm *et al.*, 1978; Table 5.5), itching, dryness and frequent rubbing of the nose (Weber *et al.*, 1976a, b). The dryness and obstruction of the nose are apparently slower to develop than other symptoms; they can give rise to mouth-breathing, with secondary complaints of a dry mouth and throat irritation. A posterior nasal drip of mucus may also provoke coughing (Weber *et al.*, 1976b).

Running of the nose was more commonly reported by non-smokers than by ex-smokers or continuing smokers (Shephard *et al.*, 1979c). In non-smokers, the symptom was commonest in the young adults, whereas in ex-smokers and continuing smokers the symptom became more common with age. In all smoking-categories, the symptom was more common in women than in men.

Special designs of body plethysmograph now permit the direct measurement of nasal resistance during passive exposure to cigarette smoke (Niinimaa *et al.*, 1979). We have not been impressed by the changes occurring over one to two hours' exposure to cigarette smoke inducing a CO concentration of 24 ppm. However, Cockcroft *et al.* (1979) have described some increase in nasal airflow resistance with exposure to cigarette smoke. Mathews (work in progress, 1980) has also observed increases of nasal airflow resistance with exposure to ammonia (concentration 100 ppm).

Other Symptoms

Suggestibility

A wide range of other symptoms are sometimes reported during passive exposure to cigarette smoke (Table 5.2), but it is difficult to rule out the influence of preconceived attitudes towards what is a visible smoke cloud and a characteristic odour.

Cameron (1972) examined the reactions of children to cigarette smoke. In a group aged 7-12 years, 76% expressed a dislike for the smoke, and only 3% said they enjoyed it. Among 13-15-year-old children, 58% expressed dislike, and 7% enjoyment. Symptoms (eye irritation, 47%; nasal irritation, 11%; headache, 12%; cough, 37%; throat trouble, nausea and other symptoms, 5-10%) were all approximately twice as frequent in those of the sample who disliked the smoke.

There seems scope for further experiments, relating the reported severity of symptoms to the hypnotic suggestibility of the individual. Nevertheless, it seems significant that almost without exception the symptoms can be traced to effects upon the eyes, the nose and the large airways, the sites of first contact between the smoke and the body; we must thus presume that the majority of complaints have some organic basis.

Locations Where Symptoms Develop

Symptoms are reported from almost every enclosed space where smoking is permitted (Shephard & LaBarre, 1976, 1978; Table 6.3). Much depends upon the daily experience of the subjects questioned. For example, at the time of the Toronto survey, 51.0% of the professional and managerial group (who used aeroplanes frequently) complained about cigarette smoke on aircraft, while only 36.2% of other occupational groups made a similar complaint. Likewise, in buses, annoyance was reported by 63.2% of those still at school, compared with 47.4% of the remainder of the sample. Some 64.4% of clerical workers reported annoyance in offices, compared with 48.7% of the remaining subjects. Finally, 40.3% of the 'housewife' group stated that they were annoyed by smoke in shops, compared with 26.7% for the rest of the sample.

The pattern of complaints is also strongly influenced by current advances in legislation and/or voluntary restriction of smoking. For instance, in 1971 (Federal Aviation Administration, 1971), 60% of non-smokers were annoyed on aircraft, whereas today the problem is

Table 6.3: Locations Where Accumulation of Cigarette Smoke is Regarded as Annoying by Non-smokers and Ex-smokers

| Location | Non-smokers | | | Ex-smokers |
	Slight nuisance %	Major annoyance %	Total %	Total %
Restaurants	33.9	33.0	72.7	64.5
Cinemas	31.4	29.2	65.9	56.9
Bars	33.1	26.8	64.8	66.6
Offices	23.4	26.1	52.5	43.0
Trains and buses	21.4	24.1	49.5	39.7
Medical facilities	16.9	22.1	41.8	32.2
Aeroplanes	16.1	19.8	39.3	39.7
Taxis	14.8	17.1	35.5	38.7
Shops	12.5	14.1	28.6	30.1

Source: Based on data from Shephard & LaBarre, 1976, 1978.

Table 6.4: Influence of Duration of Abstinence Upon Annoyance by Cigarette Smoke in Ex-smokers

| Location | Abstinence | |
	< 6 months %	> 5 years %
Restaurants	60.9	64.7
Cinemas	60.9	64.7
Bars	72.7	52.9
Offices	34.8	70.6
Trains and buses	31.8	64.7
Medical facilities	31.8	35.3
Aeroplanes	36.4	58.8
Taxis	40.9	47.1
Shops	31.8	35.3

Source: Based on data from Shephard & LaBarre, 1976, 1978.

largely controlled by cabin segregation. The proportion of subjects annoyed is all the more remarkable in view of the low CO concentrations that were recorded in the aircraft cabins (consistently < 5 ppm). In Toronto, the publication of the report of Shephard & LaBarre (1976) was shortly followed by the banning of smoking in cinemas, and the establishment of non-smoking sections in restaurants; again, a repetition of the survey would undoubtedly reflect the impact of these public health measures.

It is interesting that in the survey of Shephard & LaBarre (1976), the complaints of ex-smokers were distributed in much the same fashion as those of the non-smokers. On average, somewhat less of the ex-smokers found annoyance in a given location, but when data were classified by duration of abstinence, it was found that in those ex-smokers who had not smoked for at least five years, annoyance was as great as in the non-smokers (Table 6.4).

Odour

The olfactory receptors of the human nose are extremely sensitive. Pungent substances can be detected at concentrations of as little as one part per thousand million (Dravineks & Krotoszynsky, 1966). In general, the intensity of perception varies with the logarithm of the concentration (Fechner-Weber law;[1] Kerka & Humphreys, 1956), although perception of a given concentration is reduced by cooling of the air (Stone, 1963; Bocca & Battiston, 1964).

Of the four generally accepted modalities of smell (acid, fragrant, acrid and capric; Croker & Henderson, 1927), the acrid is the dominant component of cigarette smoke. While the odour is perceived very readily on entering a room, the nasal receptors adapt very quickly, and after a minute or so it may no longer be obvious. The threshold varies somewhat with the attitude of the individual. A convinced advocate of clean air will detect even a trace of cigarette smoke in a non-smoking area, but a person who is married to a heavy smoker may not comment on much higher smoke concentrations. Likewise, it is interesting that complaints about cigarette smoke are relatively frequent in medical facilities (Table 6.3) although the actual concentrations of smoke are relatively low (Sebben *et al.*, 1977). We may hypothesize that the sensitivity of the non-smoker is increased in such a situation by a combination of: (i) ill-health; and (ii) the conflict between the purpose of the medical facility and the voluntary contamination of its atmosphere.

Chronic smoke exposure leads to damage of the olfactory cells. Thus, a heavy smoker has a threefold increase in the smell threshold, and is more vulnerable to fatigue of the olfactory receptors (Moser, 1972; Kittel, 1976). Sensitivity to odours also diminishes with age (Kittel, 1976).

If the ceiling of cigarette smoke accumulation is to be set in terms of odour detection, a very high rate of ventilation is required. For example, in an aircraft with 15 cabin air changes per hour, the lighting of a single cigarette can be detected after only a few 'puffs'.

Note

1. Fechner, a psychophysicist, suggested sensation, R, was logarithmically related to stimulus intensity, S:

$R = c \text{ Log } S$.

See Borg, G. (1971) 'Perception of Physical Performance' in R.J. Shephard (ed.), *Frontiers of Fitness*, C.C. Thomas, Springfield, Ill., p. 281.

7 SMOKE EXPOSURE AND HEALTH

Until recently, the main focus of arguments concerning passive smoking was upon acute responses, including effects of carbon monoxide upon psychomotor function, exercise tolerance and angina threshold (see Chapter 4) and immediate changes of cardio-respiratory performance. However, there is now substantial concern that specific chemical constituents of cigarette smoke reach sufficient concentrations to cause more permanent adverse health effects both in the general population and in certain sensitive groups such as young children, the elderly and asthmatic patients.

General Population

Lung Cancer

Since tobacco smoke contains many known carcinogens (Table 1.7), there is plainly a risk that passive exposure to such agents could give rise to lung cancer in non-smokers. One recent calculation (British Medical Journal, 1978b) noted that some 75% of the benzpyrene from the smoking of a cigarette entered the atmosphere of a room in side-stream smoke. Under conditions of poor ventilation, non-smokers could inhale the equivalent of the smoking of four cigarettes over the course of a single hour; on this basis, benzpyrene from regular and heavy passive exposure would cause two cases of lung cancer per year in a group of 100,000 non-smokers. The calculation is not altogether supported by the data of Galuskinová (1964, Table 3.4), who observed benzpyrene levels of only 0.14 ng$\cdot$l^{-1} in a smoky room, compared with the 10-50 μg generated by a single cigarette. A further imponderable is that no allowance is made for the action of other carcinogens and co-carcinogens that could have an additivie or even a multiplicative effect upon risk (Stock, 1980). At the same time there seems a fallacy in assuming that active smokers escape the effects of passive smoke exposure. It could also be argued quite reasonably that in some countries much larger quantities of benzpyrene are generated by open coal fires and the burning of garden refuse, although in such circumstances the benzpyrene is rapidly dispersed into the general atmosphere, unlike the closed situation where cigarettes are commonly smoked.

Nitrosamines are a second grave concern to the non-smoker.

Table 7.1: Mortality per 100,000 Non-smoking Wives, Standardized on the Basis of Husband's Occupation or Age

| | Husband's smoking habit and occupation or age-standardized mortality | | |
Classification of husband	Non-smoker	Ex-smoker or 1–19 cigarettes per day	More than 20 cigarettes per day
Age 40–59 years	5.6	9.3	13.1
Age > 60 years	15.8	24.4	29.6
Agricultural work			
(All)	9.5	17.0	18.4
(age 40–59 years)	3.5	11.0	15.9
Other work			
(All)	9.1	10.5	17.8
(age 40–59 years)	7.2	8.1	11.1

Source: Based on data from Hirayama, 1981.

Concentrations of nitrosamines are up to 50 times higher in sidestream than in mainstream smoke, and such compounds are known to be powerful, organ-specific carcinogens; in consequence, no industrial exposure is permitted (Brunnemann *et al.*, 1977b).

A possible impact of passive smoking upon the incidence of carcinoma may be inferred from a study in Utah. Prohibition of smoking by the Mormon church greatly reduces the risk of passive exposure to cigarette smoke, and in this state the incidence of lung cancer among non-smokers is low even if they are not of the Mormon faith (Stock, 1980).

Miller (1978) examined the deaths of non-smoking women in Erie County, Pennsylvania, and noted that the wives of non-smoking husbands lived four years longer than the wives of husbands who smoked. More direct evidence on the risks of lung carcinoma was gathered by Hirayama (1981). He followed a total of 91,540 non-smoking Japanese wives over a 14-year period, classifying their standardized mortality rates for lung cancer on the basis of the smoking habits of their husbands. The risk of lung cancer increased with passive smoking among both middle-aged and older groups, irrespective of the husband's occupation, although the gradient of risk was particularly steep for women whose husbands had an agricultural occupation and were in the age range 40–59 years (Table 7.1). This presumably reflects a lesser non-domestic exposure to both cigarette smoke and other air pollutants when living in a rural environment.

The impact of the husband's smoking habits upon various causes

Table 7.2: Age and Occupation Standardized Risk Ratio for Selected
Causes of Death in Non-smoking Women, Classified by Smoking Habit
of Husband

| | Husband's smoking habit and risk ratio | | |
Cause of death	Non-smoker	Ex-smoker or 1–19 cigarettes per day	More than 20 cigarettes per day
Lung cancer	1.00	1.61	2.08
Emphysema and asthma	1.00	1.29	1.49
Cancer of cervix	1.00	1.15	1.14
Cancer of stomach	1.00	1.02	0.99
Ischaemic heart disease	1.00	0.97	1.03

Source: Based on data from Hirayama, 1981.

Table 7.3: Age and Occupation Standardized Risk Ratio for Selected
Causes of Death in Non-smoking Women, Classified by Drinking Habit
of Husband

| | Husband's drinking habit and risk ratio | | |
Cause of death	Non-drinker	Occasional or rare drinker	Daily drinker
Lung cancer	1.00	1.13	1.18
Emphysema and asthma	1.00	0.92	1.39
Cancer of cervix	1.00	0.84	0.89
Cancer of stomach	1.00	0.88	0.95
Ischaemic heart disease	1.00	1.09	0.93

Source: Based on data from Hirayama, 1981.

of death is explored in Table 7.2. While the increase of risk ratio is
highly significant for lung cancer ($P < 0.001$), none of the other risk
gradients reach the usually accepted level of statistical significance.
Nevertheless, the 49% increase in risk of death from emphysema with
passive smoking is also highly suggestive. Further, the association
between passive smoking and lung cancer seems a direct one rather than
an expression of health habits or socio-economic status, since: (i) it
is independent of occupation; and (ii) there is no significant relationship
between the husband's alcohol consumption and the wife's risk of
death from lung cancer (Table 7.3).

In Hirayama's study, the effect upon mortality was at least one-
third to half of that seen with active smoking. Further, since relatively

few Japanese women smoke (some 15% of the population), the number of women *killed* by passive exposure exceeded the number killed by active smoking.

Many smaller mammals have been subjected to passive cigarette smoke exposures over the last 10–15 years. The results of these studies are more difficult to interpret, since the doses of cigarette smoke used have often been quite high, and some varieties of experimental animal also have a high rate of spontaneous tumour formation. Lorenz *et al.* (1943) did not detect any increase of respiratory tract tumours when a group of mice were exposed to cigarette smoke for 693 hours. In contrast, Essenberg (1952) found an increase of papillary adenomas in the same strain of mice when exposures were extended to $12 \text{ h} \cdot \text{day}^{-1}$ over one year. Mühlbock (1955) observed an increased incidence of alveolar cell carcinoma (79%, versus 31% in controls) when hybrid mice were exposed to smoke for 684 days (two hours per day). Guerin (1959) exposed a colony of Wistar rats to smoke 45 minutes per day for two to six months; he also noted more tumours in experimental rats (5.1%) than in controls (2.4%). Leuchtenberger and his associates (1960b) worked with albino mice; the equivalent of eight cigarettes per day for 11 to 201 days led to adverse changes in 23 of 275 experimental animals, including basal cell hyperplasia (15 cases), atypical basal cell hyperplasia (14 cases), dysplasia (seven cases) and squamous cell metaplasia (two cases). Otto (1963) likewise observed adenomatous changes when albino mice were exposed to 12 cigarettes per day for two years, while Dontenwill & Wiebecke (1966) found that an exposure to four cigarettes per day for two years was sufficient to cause an increase of desquamative metaplasia and bronchial papillary metaplasia in a group of golden hamsters. Smoke-induced changes of DNA synthesis were described by Boren (1970), while Harris & Negroni (1967) reported enhancement of adenocarcinoma formation in a strain of mice normally resistant to tumour formation. We may thus conclude that animal experiments support the view that passive smoke exposure can induce tumour formation, although in most of the experiments cited the tumours were adenocarcinomas rather than the squamous cell carcinoma that commonly develops in human lungs.

Other Chest Diseases

Other pathological changes have been observed in the airways of animals exposed to high doses of cigarette smoke (Reece & Ball, 1972). In general, the findings resemble human chronic bronchitis and/or emphysema. Leuchtenberger *et al.* (1960a) found that 20% of mice developed severe bronchitis over exposure periods of 1–23 months. Similarly, rabbits developed focal or generalized hyperplasia of the bronchial epithelium and emphysema with two to five years of exposure (Holland *et al.*, 1963), and greyhound dogs showed emphysematous disruption of the pulmonary parenchyma after one year of exposure (Hernandez *et al.*, 1966). Inhibition of ciliary activity (see Chapter 5) makes it more difficult to rid the lungs of foreign matter, while a direct inhibition of the alveolar phagocytic cells further restricts the removal of bacteria and fine particles (Green & Carolin, 1967).

Information concerning chronic changes in man is more sketchy. The possible increase of mortality from emphysema and asthma (Table 7.2) has already been noted. Non-smokers who work in smoky offices expectorate Curschmann's spirals (bronchial casts of mucus, usually seen in chronic bronchial disorders; Stock, 1980). Moreover, non-smokers who work alongside smokers have 10–20% poorer lung function than those without such exposure, deterioration being particularly striking in tests of small airway function (White & Froeb, 1980). Similar changes have been reported in some studies of the wives of heavy smokers (Stock, 1980; Comstock, work in progress), although Bouhuys (1977) found no deterioration of pulmonary maximum expiratory flow-volume curve in households where a smoker was resident.

Children

A number of articles have suggested that young children are at particular risk from passive exposure to cigarette smoke. This seems likely on two counts: (i) young children are vulnerable both to air pollutants and respiratory pathogens because of a high respiratory minute volume per unit of body mass; and (ii) an infant or toddler has little opportunity to move away from a chain-smoking mother.

Cameron *et al.* (1969) noted a statistically significant association between parental smoking habits and the prevalence of respiratory infections in a telephone survey of children living in Detroit. Norman-Taylor & Dickinson (1972) reported similar results in a survey of 1,119 five-year-old children; respiratory infections were found in 45% of children from homes where one or both of the parents were smokers, compared with 34% of children from homes where neither of the parents smoked. A larger survey of 2,626 households confirmed the greater prevalence of acute illness (common colds, influenza, bronchitis

Table 7.4: Influence of Parental Smoking Habits on Pneumonia and Bronchitis in Children over First Five Years of Life. Subjects Classified According to Health of Parents (No Chronic Bronchitis or Winter Morning Phlegm in One or Both Parents)

Year of follow-up	Parental smoking habit and annual incidence of pneumonia or bronchitis per 100 children					
	No chronic bronchitis			One or both with bronchitis		
	Both non-smokers	One smoker	Both smokers	Both non-smokers	One smoker	Both smokers
1	7.6	10.4	15.3	10.3	14.8	23.0
2	8.1	7.1	8.7	8.3	15.5	9.2
3	6.9	10.5	7.9	8.1	9.4	11.0
4	8.0	7.5	7.6	11.1	10.8	11.6
5	6.7	5.6	3.9	14.7	9.4	10.6

Source: Based on data from Colley *et al.*, 1974.

and pneumonia) in children from homes contaminated by cigarette smoke (Cameron & Robertson, 1973). One possible explanation might be that older children were themselves smoking in households where the parents smoked; however, in the second study it was possible to demonstrate that the association persisted if the sample was restricted to children from birth to five years of age. No evidence was obtained concerning a second potential confounding variable — the lower socio-economic status of smoking parents.

In contrast, Shy *et al.* (1970) found no association between parental smoking habits and illness in the children of 871 families. Likewise, Schilling *et al.* (1977) were unable to demonstrate any relationship between parental smoking habits and respiratory symptoms or lung function test results in 816 children from 376 families. Possibly, the sample sizes were insufficient in these two studies, and possibly data were also confounded by the personal smoking of older children. More recently, Tager *et al.* (1979) have shown a crude inverse relationship between the forced expiratory flow rate and parental smoking habits, provided that the sample was restricted to children who did not smoke themselves. Results were 0.16 SD lower if one parent smoked, and 0.36 SD lower if both parents smoked.

Colley (1974) confirmed the relationship between parental smoking and childhood respiratory illness in a survey of 2,205 infants over the first five years of life (Table 7.4). Nevertheless, the study also suggested that the prevalence of respiratory infections bore a much

Table 7.5: Hospital Admission Rates per 100 Infants for First Year of Life in Relation to Maternal Smoking

Admission diagnosis	Birth weight, smoking habit of mother and hospital admission rate					
	< 3.0 kg		3.0–3.5 kg		> 3.5 kg	
	Non-smoker	Smoker	Non-smoker	Smoker	Non-smoker	Smoker
Bronchitis and pneumonia	12.3	19.2	8.2	9.6	9.0	12.1
Other diagnoses	19.9	22.6	14.5	14.6	13.3	15.2

Source: Based on data from Harlap & Davies, 1974.

stronger relationship to parental cough and phlegm production than to smoking itself. They thus argued that the children may have become infected not as a direct result of smoke exposure, but rather because active smoking led to more frequent respiratory infections in the parents. This explanation was supported by Lebowitz & Burrows (1976).

Harlap & Davies (1974) found a relationship between hospital admissions for bronchitis and pneumonia over the first year of life, and the smoking habits of the mother, as assessed during the immediately preceeding pregnancy. The association was most marked for the winter months, when smoke exposure would have been greatest. It was also most marked for infants with a low birth weight, but remained significant even for children with a normal birth weight (Table 7.5). Critics of the study have stressed that hospital admissions do not provide an infallible index of morbidity; moreover, the children of smoking mothers were more frequently admitted for injuries, poisoning, gastroenteritis, childhood infectious diseases and other diagnoses, suggesting that the children concerned had a poor overall standard of maternal care.

Further studies by Colley *et al.* (1974) and Leeder *et al.* (1976) were able to exclude some of the confounding variables. Pneumonia and bronchitis were related to parental smoking habits from birth to one year, but not from one to five years of age. Moreoever, the effect was dose-dependent (being most marked when both parents smoked, and also varying with the total daily cigarette consumption) and could be demonstrated independently of parental chest disease, social class or birth weight (Table 7.4). The most important precipitant of respiratory disease was nevertheless an attack of bronchitis or pneumonia in a sibling.

Although the main effect of cigarette smoke seems to be upon very young children, after effects are encountered in older age groups. Thus Said & Zalokar (1978) found in a survey of 4,000 Parisian high school students that the incidence of operations for excision of the tonsils and adenoids was a function of the smoking habits of the parents.

From the investigations completed to date, it remains difficult to exclude the possibility that the mother who smokes is less health conscious than the mother who does not. Nevertheless, it seems reasonable to suspect cigarette smoke as playing a direct role in the causation of respiratory disease in young children. Moreover, several recent investigators have commented on an association between maternal smoking and the sudden infant death syndrome (Bergman & Wiesner, 1976; Rhead, 1977).

Elderly Subjects

It has long been recognized that the elderly, particularly patients suffering from chronic bronchitis and emphysema, are among the individuals most likely to succumb to both particulate and gaseous contamination of the atmosphere (Ashe, 1952; Beaver, 1954). Thus, during the major London smog episodes of 1952 and 1956, a high proportion of the increase in seasonal mortality rates ('excess deaths') occurred among those who were both old and already affected by chronic chest disease.

Unfortunately, it is not very practicable to carry out experiments on sick elderly patients and, perhaps for this reason, there do not seem to have been any experimental or epidemiological studies on the tolerance of such subjects to passive cigarette smoke exposure.

Asthmatic Patients

Allergenic Properties of Tobacco Smoke

There is little question that some tobacco field workers become allergic to the plants they are harvesting, but there is more controversy concerning the possibility of developing an allergy to cigarette smoke. Some authorities maintain that there is as yet no evidence of a true allergic reaction (in the sense that exposure to tobacco smoke has not yet been shown to induce the formation of a unique serum antibody).

Much of the early work on 'tobacco allergy' was based upon skin testing (Justus & Adams, 1976), and it remains uncertain how far the existence of skin reactions to tobacco extracts can be equated with the response of the respiratory tract to cigarette smoke (Taylor, 1974). Moreover, not all investigators took care to distinguish between irritation of the skin and a true allergic reaction. Tests were rarely conducted in double-blind fashion, and allergy was sometimes diagnosed in the absence of clinical symptoms. On other occasions, patients were not in a truly, asymptomatic state, and the tobacco smoke may have played a secondary role, aggravating responses to some other allergen.

Brown (1923) found that 1% of asthmatic patients had positive skin reactions to tobacco leaf extracts, and some subsequent investigators claimed that the skin reaction could be transferred in a passive fashion to normal control subjects (Harvaky, 1939; Peshkin & Landay, 1939; Lima & Rocha, 1949; Becker & Dubin, 1977). However, other workers were unable to confirm these observations (Sulzberger, 1933; Chobot, 1934; Trasoff *et al.*, 1936; Westcott & Wright, 1938). Some authors also suggested that extracts of tobacco smoke were capable of reacting with human antibodies, leading to immediate skin reactions (Pipes, 1945; Becker & Dubin, 1977) and delayed skin reactions (Sulzberger, 1933).

The basis of any allergic reaction could be the natural proteins of the tobacco leaf or contaminants of the plant, including bacteria, fungi, insecticides and other allergens (such as ragweed pollen). The tobacco leaf contains several protein/carbohydrate complexes of molecular weight 10,000 to 60,000 that are capable of stimulating antibody formation, and precipitating human antisera (Chu *et al.*, 1970; Kreis *et al.*, 1970; Panayotopoulos *et al.*, 1974). According to Becker & Dubin (1977), the natural glycoproteins of tobacco give rise to immediate skin reactions in about one-third of individuals.

Skin Reactions in Asthmatic Patients

Fontana *et al.* (1959) found that 64% of 'allergic' children gave positive skin reactions to tobacco leaf extract, as compared with only 6% of controls. Others set reactions at 12% of asthmatic patients (Rosen, 1954), 15% of 'allergic' individuals (Speer, 1968) and 13% of 'allergic' individuals (Pipes, 1945). In the last study, 10% of patients also complained of exacerbation of symptoms when exposed to tobacco smoke.

We may conclude that tobacco extracts can yield skin reactions, but it is not clear how far the apparently specific response of the asthmatic subject reflects an irritant effect upon capillary membranes that have already been pathologically sensitized by allergic reactions to other allergens. Further, the link between skin sensitivity and respiratory tract reactions is tenuous (Taylor, 1974).

Respiratory Tract Reactions

Many of the irritant effects of tobacco smoke could on casual inspection be interpreted as having an allergic basis. Thus Speer (1968) found that in a sample of 250 non-allergic and non-smoking individuals, passive exposure to cigarette smoke induced nasal symptoms such as sneezing and itchiness in 29%, cough in 25%, headache in 33% and eye irritation in 70% of subjects. Nasal symptoms, headache, cough, sore throat and nausea were all more common in 191 'allergic' individuals (patients with nasal allergy, asthma or allergic headache) than in the non-allergic group. Twenty-one of the 191 'allergic' subjects gave a positive skin reaction to a tobacco scratch test, but these individuals did not develop a particularly severe respiratory tract reaction to the cigarette smoke exposure.

Broder *et al.* (1974) suggested that most symptoms of allergic rhinitis could be traced to specific allergens and, in their view, neither smoking nor passive exposure to cigarette smoke made a major contribution to this disorder.

Certainly, some reports of tobacco sensitivity are only anecdotal. Thus Blue (1970) described a heavy smoker who developed frequent attacks of asthma during the winter months. After giving up smoking, the asthmatic symptoms disappeared. Savel (1970) described eight non-smokers with hypersensitivity to tobacco smoke. All had an 'allergic' history and developed immediate respiratory discomfort on being exposed to cigarette smoke. Zussman (1970) studied 16 atopic patients with allergic reactions to pollen, food or drugs. All developed nasal, ocular and bronchial symptoms during passive smoking, but these symptoms disappeared 15–20 minutes after the exposure was terminated.

Shephard *et al.* (1979c) found that rather more smokers than non-smokers reported wheezing during passive smoking (Table 7.6). In both ex-smokers and continuing smokers, the frequency of wheezing was greater in older subjects, and in the continuing smokers, the likelihood of a wheezing response was also related to cigarette consumption. Irrespective of smoking habits, wheezing was twice as common in asthmatics (25%) as in non-asthmatics (12%). We may thus suspect that both smoking-induced chest disease and asthma increased the sensitivity of the individual to the irritant effects of the smoke. However, it remains arguable that the response was basically non-allergic in nature,

Table 7.6: Subjective Reactions Caused by Passive Exposure to
Cigarette Smoke

Smoking habit	Wheezing %	Rhinorrhoea %
Non-smoker	11.0	19.3
Ex-smoker	9.4	11.5
Smoker	15.0	6.1

Source: Based on data from Shephard *et al.* 1979c.

particularly as smokers and ex-smokers were less liable to rhinorrhoea than their non-smoking counterparts.

Zussman (1974) reported that 16% of adults were clinically irritated by tobacco smoke. Thirteen of 16 such patients claimed benefit from desensitization injections. Nevertheless, the interpretation of these observations is problematical, since the antigens used were a complex mixture of tobacco extracts and house dusts.

O'Connell & Logan (1974) interviewed 400 asthmatic and 228 control children, finding little difference of parental smoking habits between the two groups. Nevertheless, tobacco smoke was reported as aggravating asthma in 53% of all asthmatic children, and in 67% of those whose parents smoked, compared with 11% of control subjects. Symptoms improved in 18 of 20 children where the parents stopped smoking, but in only four of 15 children where the parents continued to smoke.

Rosen & Levy (1950) described an infant who developed an asthmatic reaction to cigarette smoke; in this report, an antibody to tobacco extract was reportedly documented. One recent Swedish report (Stahle & Tibbling, 1978) has also described provocation of asthmatic attacks in 21% of patients by the inhalation of tobacco extracts, but it is less certain that the compounds responsible are found in cigarette smoke.

We may conclude that there is good evidence that tobacco smoke is more irritant to the respiratory tract of an asthmatic patient than it is to a normal individual. However, in most of the experiments cited, true allergens have not been clearly demonstrated. As with the skin reactions discussed above, the bronchial spasm may be no more than an exaggerated response to irritants in a system made reactive by previous exposure to other allergens.

Table 7.7: Symptoms Anticipated and Those Reported by Asthmatic Non-smokers Compared to Response of Non-asthmatic Subjects. Two Hours' Passive Exposure to Cigarette Smoke

Symptom	Per cent of asthmatics anticipating symptom	Per cent reporting symptom		Average severity (0 = absent, 5 = incapacitating)
		Normal subjects	Asthmatic subjects	Asthmatic subjects
Headache	8	15	21	0.4
Stinging eyes	31	95	93	1.9
Running nose or stuffiness	46	55	29	0.6
Phlegm	8	40	21	0.4
Wheezing	31	10	38	0.8
Shortness of breath	23	15	21	0.5
Tightness in chest	23	5	43	0.5
Cough	46	45	36	0.6
Sore throat	16	—	14	0.3
Nausea	8	10	0	0
Dizziness	16	10	0	0

Source: Based on data from Shephard *et al.*, 1979b.

Table 7.8: Effects of Two Hours' Passive Exposure to Cigarette Smoke Upon Static Lung Volumes of Asthmatic Patients. All Results Expressed as Per Cent of Corresponding Sham Exposure Value

Variable	Immediate exposure	Two-hour exposure
Vital capacity	99.8	98.0
Residual volume	109.6	93.0
Functional residual capacity	103.9	95.2
Total lung capacity	103.5[a]	96.5[b]

Notes: a. $P < 0.01$.
    b. $P < 0.02$.
Source: Based on data from Shephard *et al.*, 1979b.

Table 7.9: Effects of Two-hour Passive Exposure to Cigarette Smoke Upon Dynamic Lung Volumes of Asthmatic Patients. All Results Expressed as Per Cent of Corresponding Sham Exposure Value

Variable	Immediate exposure	1-hour exposure	2-hour exposure
Forced vital capacity	101.3	100.1	100.6
One second forced expiratory volume	103.1	99.2	101.4
Maximum expiratory flow at 50% of vital capacity	97.6	94.1	99.6
Maximum expiratory flow at 25% of vital capacity	101.6	86.6	124.8

Source: Based on data from Shephard *et al.* 1979b.

Table 7.10: Changes of Lung Volumes in Asthmatic Subjects Reporting a Sensitivity to Cigarette Smoke, Compared with Changes in the Remainder of the Group. Values after Two-hour Experimental Exposure Expressed as Per Cent of Corresponding Sham Exposure Value

Variable	Sensitive subjects	Other subjects
Vital capacity	101	97
Residual volume	85	97
Functional residual capacity	92	96
Total lung capacity	97	96
Forced vital capacity	100	101
One second forced expiratory volume	107[a]	99
Maximum expiratory flow at 50% of vital capacity	103	97
Maximum expiratory flow at 25% of vital capacity	100	99

Note: a. $P < 0.05$.
Source: Based on data from Shephard *et al.*, 1979b.

Experimental Exposure of Asthmatics

Shephard *et al.* (1979b) carried out a series of experimental cigarette smoke exposures on 14 asthmatic non-smokers. The symptoms reported while in the chamber (Table 7.7) were somewhat different from what had been anticipated by the subjects. However, it is significant that, as in healthy individuals, the most frequent and most severe complaint was of eye irritation rather than chest tightness or wheezing; although eye symptoms were anticipated by only 31% of subjects, they were actually reported by 93% of the sample. The most commonly anticipated complaints were cough and nasal discharge or stuffiness. The asthmatic triad of wheezing, shortness of breath and tightness in the chest developed a little more frequently than the patients had anticipated, and it is worth comment that such symptoms were more frequent than in non-asthmatic subjects exposed to the same environment. Nevertheless, in most of the asthmatics who developed respiratory symptoms, these were not particularly severe or incapacitating.

At the beginning of experimental exposure, the static lung volumes of the asthmatic sample were much as in the corresponding sham exposure, with the exception that total lung capacity showed a small increase, possibly an emotional reaction as the polluted atmosphere was first encountered (Tables 7.8 and 7.9).

Data were analyzed separately for the four subjects who anticipated wheezing during smoke exposure (Table 7.10). Static lung volumes showed an insignificantly greater decline in the sensitive subjects. The only significant difference ($P < 0.05$) was a small increase of forced expiratory flow rate in those claiming sensitivity to cigarette smoke. It is possible that this sub-group was more nervous in the exposure chamber, and thus developed some catecholamine-induced bronchodilatation, although the increase of heart rate (about 4% above the corresponding sham exposure value) was quite small even in this sub-group.

We may conclude that in terms of both symptoms and objective signs of 'gas-trapping', asthmatics as a class have a greater than normal reaction to cigarette smoke. On the other hand, the experimental data do not support the view that any sub-group of asthmatic patients has an unusual sensitivity to the smoke. The findings are more in keeping with irritation of sensitized airways than with a specific allergic reaction.

8 ATTITUDES TO CIGARETTE SMOKE ACCUMULATION

Attitudes towards the accumulation of cigarette smoke in public places have undergone a substantial change over the past ten years. Both smokers and non-smokers now find heavy contamination of the atmosphere unacceptable. Documentation of such attitudes is an important preliminary step on the road to cleaner air, whether the remedy be sought in terms of legislation, voluntary controls or engineering solutions such as the improved ventilation of public facilities.

General Public

Overall Attitudes to Air Contamination

Two studies from Toronto have examined the attitudes of the general public as encountered in areas such as shopping centres (Baker & MacKendrick, 1976; Shephard & LaBarre, 1976, 1978). At the time of these studies (the mid-1970s), industry was the main perceived culprit responsible for air pollution in heavily contaminated areas of the city. Vehicles and refineries were less commonly blamed, while smoking and the emissions from domestic furnaces were accused relatively infrequently (Table 8.1). In residential areas of the city, vehicles were seen as the main polluters, with a substantial minority of subjects placing prime blame upon the domestic furnace and industry. Cigarette smoking was given more weight in residential than in polluted areas of the city, but nevertheless it was rarely regarded as the prime pollutant.

When the data were reclassified by smoking habits (Table 8.2), conclusions were generally similar, although the proportion identifying tobacco smoke as the major problem was somewhat greater among non-smokers and ex-smokers than among continuing smokers. When data were classified on an age basis, the young were found to be more critical of industry, while older subjects criticized vehicles (Table 8.3). More importantly in our present context, the oldest age group had the most complaints about passive smoking. Among possible explanations we may note: (i) the 60–80-year-old group often no longer live in their own homes — there is thus unaccustomed exposure to cigarette smoke and little opportunity to escape; (ii) the elderly move mainly in residential sections of the city and thus have little experience of other

Table 8.1: Greatest Perceived Source of Pollution in Heavily
Contaminated and in Residential Areas of Toronto

Prime source of pollution	Heavily polluted areas (% of subjects)	Residential areas (% of subjects)
Industry	57.2	12.3
Vehicles	24.0	65.0
Refineries (petrol, lead, etc.)	14.4	2.8
Domestic furnace	1.2	15.1
Smoking	3.1	4.7

Source: Based on data from Shephard & LaBarre, 1976, 1978.

Table 8.2: Percentage of Subjects Perceiving Smoking as Prime Source
of Pollution in Heavily Contaminated and in Residential Areas of
Toronto (Subjects Classified by Smoking Habits)

Smoking habits of subjects	Heavily polluted areas (% of subjects)	Residential areas (% of subjects)
Non-smoker	3.5	6.3
Ex-smoker	4.1	4.1
Cigarette smoker		
(< 5 cigarettes/day)	2.5	1.7
(> 5 cigarettes/day)	2.8	4.3
Pipe or cigar	0.0	0.0

Source: Based on data from Shephard & LaBarre, 1976, 1978.

Table 8.3: Percentage of Subjects Perceiving Smoking as Prime Source
of Pollution in Heavily Contaminated and in Residential Areas of
Toronto (Subjects Classified by Age)

Age of subjects	Heavily polluted areas		Residential areas	
	% of men	% of women	% of men	% of women
10–20 years	2.2	0.0	4.5	1.2
20–40	4.1	3.2	3.5	6.5
40–60	4.3	2.2	5.8	7.8
60–80	12.0	7.7	8.0	15.4

Source: Based on data from Shephard & LaBarre, 1976, 1978.

Table 8.4: Influence of Occupational Status Upon Concern Regarding Air Pollution (for Subjects in Labour Force)

Level of concern	Occupational category		
	Professional & managerial	Clerical & sales	Manual
High	37.3	35.9	26.1
Average	54.9	53.2	61.1
Low	7.8	10.8	12.9

Source: Based on data from Shephard & LaBarre, 1976, 1978.

Table 8.5: Influence of Age Upon Concern Regarding Air Pollution

Age of subjects	Percent with high level of concern	
	Men	Women
10–20 years	23.9	20.4
20–40	28.9	28.0
40–60	46.4	53.3
60–80	52.0	53.8

Source: Based on data from Shephard & LaBarre, 1976, 1978.

Table 8.6: Influence of Concern about Air Pollution upon Voting Habits

Voting habit	Concern about air pollution		
	High %	Average %	Low %
Always or usually vote	69.9	51.4	36.9
Rarely or never vote	30.1	48.6	63.1

Source: Based on data from Shephard & LaBarre, 1976, 1978.

types of urban air pollution; and (iii) failing vision may be particularly vulnerable to the effects of eye irritants (see Chapter 6).

Concern about air pollution was somewhat greater in high than in low status occupational groups (Table 8.4). In contrast with an earlier report by Harvey *et al.* (1974), Shephard & LaBarre (1976, 1978) found that concern increased somewhat as subjects became older (Table 8.5).

The sample questioned was not exceptional in terms of political activism. Excluding students, 60% of the group always or usually voted. There was the anticipated social gradient among those exercising their franchise (82% of professional and managerial class, 52% of clerical and sales workers and 51% of manual workers). Exercise of the franchise was also influenced by smoking habits (95% of pipe and cigar smokers, 60% of non-smokers, 55% of ex-smokers and 49% of continuing cigarette smokers). Voting habits were strongly influenced by concern about air pollution (Table 8.6).

Specific Attitudes Towards Cigarette Smoke

The attitude towards a municipal politican who was prepared to enact 'tougher' legislation to control smoking in public places was strongly supportive, irrespective of occupational category. Classifying data by smoking habits, 90.7% of non-smokers would vote for such a candidate and, more surprisingly, 79.6% of ex-smokers, 79.0% of pipe or cigar smokers, 79.0% of light cigarette smokers and 67.9% of heavy cigarette smokers offered their support (Table 8.7); even among this last category, less than 15% were opposed to such legislation.

As might be anticipated, there was a sharp gradient of opinion with concern about air pollution in general (Table 8.8). Support for control legislation was shown by 89% of those with a high level of concern, 79% of those with average concern and 59% of those with a low level of concern. Support for controls was also related to knowledge of the health effects of smoking (Table 8.9), and to more general exercise of the political franchise (Table 8.10), tending to increase with the age of the subject (Table 8.11).

Only a small minority of non-smokers (11.6%) said that they were unaffected by passive exposure to cigarette smoke. Responses were divided rather evenly between those who regarded smoke accumulation as a nuisance (46.8%) and those who thought that it had a major effect upon their health (41.6%), although more of the older women made this last category of response. Ex-smokers apparently were less conscious of cigarette smoke; 37.6% were unaffected by passive exposure and only 23.6% reported a major effect upon their health.

Accumulation of cigarette smoke was apparently tolerated less well at the office than at home. Some 38% of non-smokers had smoking room-mates, and 55% of this sample believed that their health was
d by the passive smoke exposure. About 51% of non-smokers
d to tobacco smoke at work, and 66% of this sample
their health was adversely affected in consequence.

Table 8.7: Attitudes Towards a Municipal Politician who was Prepared
to Enact 'Tougher' Legislation to Control Smoking in Public Places
(Subjects Classified by Smoking Habits)

Attitude towards politician	Non-smoker	Ex-smoker	Continuing smoker <5 cigs/day	>5 cigs/day	Pipe or cigar smoker
Strongly support	62.1	48.0	29.4	24.7	47.4
Some support	28.6	31.6	49.6	43.2	31.6
	90.7	*79.6*	*79.0*	*67.9*	*79.0*
Indifferent	7.2	12.2	10.1	17.3	10.5
Opposed	2.1	8.2	10.9	14.8	10.5

Source: Based on data from Shephard & LaBarre, 1976, 1978.

Table 8.8: Attitudes Towards a Municipal Politician who was
Prepared to Enact 'Tougher' Legislation to Control Smoking in Public
Places (Subjects Classified by Concern about Air Pollution)

Attitude towards politician	Concern about air pollution High %	Average %	Low %
Strongly support	74.3	31.9	18.9
Some support	15.0	47.3	39.6
	89.3	*79.2*	*58.5*
Indifferent	5.3	13.0	22.5
Opposed	5.3	7.8	18.9

Source: Based on data from Shephard & LaBarre, 1976, 1978.

Some 73% of non-smokers had seen material on the health hazards of passive exposure to cigarette smoke. The proportion with such knowledge rose to more than 90% among those non-smokers who were over 40 years of age. Ex-smokers were somewhat less well-informed on the dangers of passive smoking, only 62% of them having seen such information. Among the continuing smokers, 24% were unaware of the risks of passive smoking, and a further 9% had read such reports, but did not believe them. Nevertheless, a gratifying 67% of smokers knew of the problem and were concerned about the effects of 'second-hand' smoke upon the non-smoker. The percentage of concerned smokers increased with age, from 60% (male) and 64% (female) in the age group 10-20 years, to 83% (male) and 84% (female) in those aged 60-80 years.

Table 8.9: Influence of Knowledge of Health Effects of Smoking Upon Attitude Towards a Politician Willing to Enact 'Tougher' Legislation to Control Smoking in Public Places

Attitude towards politician	Lung cancer		'Scientists have proven that smoking causes . . .' Chronic chest disease		Coronary disease		Problem to unborn babies	
	Yes %	No %	Yes %	No %	Yes %	No %	Yes %	No %
Strongly support	46.2	35.9	50.9	30.4	55.6	32.5	52.4	34.7
Some support	36.8	35.5	32.5	43.6	29.5	43.0	31.8	41.2
83.0	*71.4*	*83.4*	*74.0*	*85.1*	*75.5*	*84.2*	*75.9*	
Indifferent	9.7	17.5	9.1	16.3	8.3	14.8	8.6	14.8
Opposed	7.3	11.2	7.4	9.7	6.7	9.7	7.2	9.3

Source: Based on data from Shephard & LaBarre, 1976, 1978.

Table 8.10: Influence of Voting Habits Upon Attitude Towards a
Politician Willing to Enact 'Tougher' Legislation to Control Smoking
in Public Places

Attitude towards politician	Voting habit			
	Always vote %	Usually vote %	Rarely vote %	Never vote %
Strongly support	60.8	37.6	35.3	30.9
Some support	25.3	42.8	41.2	43.9
	86.1	*80.4*	*76.5*	*74.8*
Indifferent	6.6	12.1	14.7	15.9
Opposed	7.3	7.5	8.8	9.3

Source: Based on data from Shephard & LaBarre, 1976, 1978.

Locations where non-smokers and ex-smokers reported annoyance
have already been discussed (see Chapter 6). The responses depend in
part upon the daily experience of individual subjects, and the figures
cited are thus minimum estimates of annoyance in a specific situation;
for instance, that proportion of subjects who do not travel by air are
unlikely to report annoyance on aircraft (Table 8.12). Nevertheless,
in most situations the proportion of smokers who regarded second-hand
smoke as potentially annoying was at least as great as the proportion of
non-smokers who found it so.

Attitudes Towards Control of Smoking

About half of both non-smokers and ex-smokers thought that the main
responsibility for the control of cigarette smoke accumulation lay with
the general public (Table 8.13). The role of both government (G) and
public health workers (P) was more commonly accorded prime responsibility by those who found smoke a nuisance (27.4%, G; 19.2%, P)
or a hazard to health (27.9%, G; 18.6%, P) than by those who were
unaffected (19.6%, G; 3.9%, P). Similar trends were shown by those
aware of the hazards of passive smoking (28.7%, G; 17.4%, P) and those
liable to various types of allergy (25.9%, G; 11.8%, P).

The allocation of prime responsibility in general varied little with
the location where the non-smoker was affected, the one exception
being shops (where 24.6% accorded responsibility to public health
workers, and 18.3% to government). (Municipal regulations in
Metropolitan Toronto prohibit smoking in major food stores, and
this regulation is enforced by public health departments.)

Control measures other than prohibition of smoking (segregated
accommodation and/or increased ventilation) inevitably carry some

Table 8.11: Influence of Age and Sex Upon Support of a Politician Willing to Enact 'Tougher' Legislation to Control Smoking in Public Places

Attitude towards politician	Male subjects				Female subjects			
	10–20 yrs %	20–40 yrs %	40–60 yrs %	60–80 yrs %	10–20 yrs %	20–40 yrs %	40–60 yrs %	60–80 yrs %
Strongly support	27.6	41.2	56.5	60.0	29.3	53.8	58.2	76.9
Some support	44.0	36.2	29.0	28.0	46.1	32.8	31.9	3.8
71.6	*71.6*	*77.4*	*85.5*	*88.0*	*75.4*	*86.6*	*90.1*	*80.7*
Indifferent	14.2	13.2	8.7	8.0	15.0	7.5	6.6	19.2
Opposed	14.2	9.4	5.8	4.0	9.6	5.9	3.3	0

Source: Based on data from Shephard & LaBarre, 1976, 1978.

Table 8.12: Locations Where an Accumulation of Cigarette Smoke is Annoying to Non-smokers (as Perceived by a Sample of 483 Smokers)

Location	Per cent of sample perceiving potential for annoyance
Aeroplanes	54.3
Trains and buses	60.1
Taxis	51.4
Restaurants	65.7
Bars	56.8
Cinemas	58.6
Offices	54.5
Shops	40.3
Medical facilities	66.7

Source: Based on data from Shephard & LaBarre, 1976, 1978.

Table 8.13: Main Responsibility for Control of Cigarette Smoke Accumulation (Data Classified by Smoking Habits of Subjects)

Site of responsibility	Non-smokers %	Ex-smokers %
Government	26.6	12.9
Public health workers	17.3	32.2
Ventilating engineers	1.6	1.1
General public	50.7	49.5
Other	3.6	3.2

Source: Based on results from Shephard & LaBarre, 1976, 1978.

Table 8.14: Tolerance of Increased Costs for Control of Tobacco Smoke by Segregation and/or Improved Ventilation (Data Classified by Smoking Habits of Subjects)

Cost tolerated	Non-smokers %	Ex-smokers %	Continuing smokers %
None	36.6	29.0	67.8
5%	6.8	5.4	10.1
10%	3.9	4.3	7.4
> 10%	1.8	4.3	4.5
	12.5	*14.0*	*22.0*
Borne by smoker	50.5	55.9	9.5[a]

Note: a. To be borne by non-smoker.
Source: Based on results from Shephard & LaBarre, 1976, 1978.

cost to the consumer. Subjects were asked what increase in costs (fares, cinema admission prices and so on) that they would tolerate in order to control smoke accumulation (Table 8.14). The majority of non-smokers believed that any additional costs should be borne by the continuing smokers. Ex-smokers concurred with this opinion. Very few of the smokers felt that the non-smokers should bear the costs of their habit, but less than a quarter were themselves prepared to pay more to ensure cleaner air for the non-smoker. The younger smokers were somewhat more willing to spend money in this direction than were those over the age of 40 years. The desire of non-smokers to see the added costs borne by the smoker was greater if health was affected by the smoking of a room-mate (60%), than where such smoking had no effect (47%) or the room-mate did not smoke (48%). Exposure to tobacco smoke at work had a similar influence; where occupational exposure to cigarette smoke was thought to affect health, 59% of subjects felt the smoker should bear the cost, compared with 44% of subjects who did not perceive any health effect from exposure at work and 47% of subjects where there was no exposure at work. Knowledge of the health effects of passive smoking was a further factor causing redirection of financial responsibility towards the smokers (53% as opposed to 44%). Among the smokers, the willingness to pay added costs to continue their habit increased from 21% in the lightest smokers (< 5 cigarettes per day) to 38% in the heaviest smokers (> 40 cigarettes per day). However, there was also an increase in the proportion suggesting that non-smokers should bear the costs (from 5% in the lightest smokers to 15% in those smoking 20–40 cigarettes per day and 13% in those smoking more than 40 cigarettes per day). The willingness to meet added costs was similar in those wishing to stop smoking and in those who did not wish to stop, but the respective proportions wishing the costs to be borne by the non-smoker were 7% and 14%.

Continuing smokers were asked whether it was reasonable that they should be asked politely to stop smoking. Some 94% of respondents accepted such action in a non-smoking area, and 88% also accepted it for other enclosed areas.

The majority of continuing smokers either favoured (37%) or were indifferent (48%) to the establishment of more non-smoking areas in public places (Table 8.15). Those regarding such a move as an intrusion upon their personal liberty were more numerous among those who did not wish to give up smoking (23%) than among those who had some wish to stop their addiction (9%).

Table 8.15: Attitudes of 483 Smokers to more Non-smoking Areas in Public Facilities, Classified by Reasons for Wishing to Stop Smoking

| Attitude to more non-smoking areas | Future health % | Pressure from relative % | Reason for wanting to stop | | | | Don't wish to stop % |
			Doctor's advice %	Symptoms %	Example to children %	Other %	
Help me to give up smoking	53.2	54.5	44.4	31.2	25.0	30.6	49.7
Indifferent	40.3	27.3	33.3	53.2	50.0	55.1	49.7
Intrusion on liberty	6.5	18.2	22.2	15.6	25.0	13.3	19.9

Source: Based on data from Shephard & LaBarre, 1976, 1978.

9 POSSIBLE REMEDIES

Given that currently occurring passive exposures to cigarette smoke present a significant hazard to health, possible options include an improvement of ventilation, voluntary restrictions upon the usage of cigarettes and legislation to enforce no-smoking zones.

Ventilation

Importance of Ventilation

Our survey of bars and restaurants (Sebben *et al.*, 1977) suggested that cigarette smoke accumulated mainly in rooms that were poorly ventilated. Given a modern and efficient ventilation system, carbon monoxide concentrations could apparently be held below 10 ppm, even when such premises were occupied by a high proportion of smokers. Other authors, also, have indicated that inadequate ventilation is the prime reason for a build-up of various smoke constituents in ambient air.

Natural and Dilution Ventilation

The natural ventilation of a room is not a particularly satisfactory means of regulating pollution, since the extent of such ventilation varies with wind pressure, wind direction, solar radiation, local convection currents and the personal whim of the room occupants with respect to the opening and closing of windows and doors. Dilution ventilation implies the use of some mechanical system such as a fan or vehicle movement to force fresh air into or extract stale air from the enclosed space. The minimum requirement to avoid an accumulation of body odours is about 0.4 m^3 of fresh air per person per minute. Given a room volume of 40 m^3, this amounts to one air change per person every 100 minutes, or if there are four occupants about 2.5 air changes per hour (Roach, 1973). If heavy physical work is to be performed, a doubling of this standard is recommended.

Pollution Levels

Calculations of ventilation per room occupant are not particularly satisfactory for regulating the accumulation of cigarette smoke, since not all of the occupants are smokers and not all of the smokers will be smoking. A more logical approach is to base calculations on the weight of tobacco being burnt, with appropriate assumptions concerning the relative proportions of mainstream and sidestream smoke and retention of mainstream smoke constituents (Thayer, 1981).

The concentration of smoke C_s (in ppm) at a distance A from a cigarette can be calculated using a simple formula for pollution of a hemisphere:

$$C_s = EB^2/VA^2$$

where E is the rate of emission of the pollutant ($ml \cdot sec^{-1}$), A is the distance from the cigarette (m), V is the ventilation ($m^3 \cdot sec^{-1}$), and B is the radius of the hemisphere (m). The surface of the hemisphere is $2\pi B^2$. Thus, if V is expressed as linear ventilation ($m^3 \cdot sec^{-1}$ per m^2, or $m \cdot sec^{-1}$) we may write:

$$C_s = 0.16\, E/VA^2$$

Let us suppose that the room under study has a cross section of 8 m^2 in the direction of air extraction. If the air supply is 1.6 $m^3 \cdot min^{-1}$, then $V = 0.2$ $m \cdot min^{-1}$, or 0.0033 $m \cdot sec^{-1}$. The carbon monoxide emitted by a cigarette is about 0.13 $ml \cdot sec^{-1}$, and at a distance of 1 metre from the cigarette:

$$C_s = 0.16 \times 0.13/3.3 \times 10^{-3} \times 1^2 = 6.3\ \text{ppm}$$

If several cigarettes are being smoked simultaneously, the likely distribution of gas concentrations can be calculated graphically by adding estimates for individual hemispheres. With more than five sources the pollution becomes essentially uniform and proportional to the 'dilution ratio' ($C_s = E/V$, where E is the total emission into the room, expressed in $ml \cdot sec^{-1}$, and V is the ventilation, expressed in $m^3 \cdot sec^{-1}$). Let us suppose that six cigarettes are burning; E is then 0.78 $ml \cdot sec^{-1}$, and assuming V is unchanged at 1.6 $m^3 \cdot min^{-1}$ or 0.026 $m^3 \cdot sec^{-1}$, we find:

$$C_s = 0.78/0.026 = 30\ \text{ppm}$$

Such figures coincide closely with the range of carbon monoxide concentrations we have observed in areas where smoking is permitted (Sebben *et al.*, 1977). Similar calculations can be made for suspended particulate matter. With a solitary smoker, the emission rate is about 1.5 mg·min^{-1}, or 0.025 mg·sec^{-1}, and if C_s is expressed in mg·m^{-3}, then:

$$C_s = 0.16 \times 0.025/3.3 \times 10^{-3} \times 1^2 = 1.2 \text{ mg·m}^{-3}$$

Again, these estimates of particulate density coincide well with experimental measurements (Table 3.3).

Ventilation Standards

The total respiratory volume of a typical subject is about 15 m^3 per 24-hour day, or 5 m^3 per working day of eight hours. From the viewpoint of danger to health, it may be reasonable to set the ceiling for passive exposure to cigarette smoke at the equivalent of the active smoking of one cigarette per day. This implies inhaling no more than 17 mg of particulate matter per day. The proposed ventilation of 1.6 m^3·min^{-1} is thus just about sufficient to accommodate a spouse who is living with a chain-smoking partner. The exposure is calculated as concentration $\times$ respiratory volume (1.2 $\times$ 15 = 18 mg particulate matter per day). If six occupants of a house or office were chain smokers, the exposure of the non-smoker (5.8 $\times$ 15 = 87 mg of particulate matter per day, 5.1 cigarette equivalents) would plainly be excessive; indeed, even an occupational exposure (5.8 $\times$ 5 = 29 mg of particulate matter, 1.7 cigarette equivalents per day) would cause some concern. Moreover, the air pollutants generated by a single smoker (CO = 6.3 ppm; particulates 1.2 mg·m^{-3}) are sufficient to create smell, irritation of the eyes and annoyance. According to Johansson & Ronge (1966), a ventilation of 50 m^3·h^{-1} is needed for every cigarette smoked in order to avoid an accumulation of tobacco odours. Given occupancy of a room by a chain-smoker (four cigarettes per hour), a ventilation of 3.3 m^3·min^{-1} would thus be required.

Thayer (1981) adopted a six-point irritation index, ranging from 0 (imperceptible) to 5 (intolerable). Data were surprisingly similar for smokers and non-smokers. Moreover, if the average judgement of a given atmosphere was '2' (acceptable ventilation), this view was accepted by 66% of room occupants; the ventilation thus calculated had to be approximately doubled to satisfy 80% of the room occupants. Other possible variables included the temperature and humidity of the air (Kerka & Humphreys, 1956), other pollutants (for instance, smog versus negative ions; Frey, 1968; Soyka & Edmonds, 1977), and the nature of the room furnishings (particularly their capacity to absorb smoke constituents). The increase of carbon monoxide concentration corresponding to 80% satisfaction with ventilation was a little over 3 ppm, while the necessary ventilation for a single smoker, as calculated from the irritation index, was 2 $m^3 \cdot min^{-1}$ for 66% satisfaction and 4 $m^3 \cdot min^{-1}$ for 80% satisfaction of room occupants.

It should be stressed that in older European buildings, heated by coal fires, the natural ventilation substantially exceeds these standards. Frazer & Stallybrass (1948) set the ventilation induced by a British coal fire at 50 to 100 $m^3 \cdot min^{-1}$; given a wall area of 40 m^2 for a typical house, this would amount to a linear velocity of 1.25-2.5 $m \cdot min^{-1}$, six to twelve times the minimal ventilation discussed above. However, such vigorous air currents are unlikely in modern North American homes, well-insulated against the heat of summer and the rigours of winter.

Energy Costs

The excess energy cost associated with the clearance of cigarette smoke from the air can be calculated from the difference between the normal minimal ventilatory requirement (0.4 $m^3 \cdot min^{-1}$ per person) and that required to avoid an excessive accumulation of cigarette smoke. The worst case might be a room occupied by six smokers and one non-smoker. The minimum ventilation to dispel body odours is 2.8 $m^3 \cdot min^{-1}$, but that needed to hold the exposure of the non-smoker to one cigarette per day is 8.2 $m^3 \cdot min^{-1}$, an excess of 5.4 $m^3 \cdot min^{-1}$. The temperature differential $\Delta°C$ can be related to ventilation using the formula (Roach, 1973):

$$\Delta°C = 0.0144\, H/V$$

where H is the heat output in $kJ \cdot min^{-1}$ and V is the volume of ventilation measured in $m^3 \cdot sec^{-1}$. If the temperature differential between the room and the environment is 40°C, as may occur on a severe winter day:

$$40 = 0.0144\, H/0.09$$

so that $H = 250$ $kJ \cdot min^{-1}$ or 4.16 kW. In a more typical winter day, the temperature differential is 20°C, and the energy cost is 2 kW. A similar energy usage is incurred for refrigeration in summer.

It is hardly surprising that some bars and restaurants have allowed cigarette smoke to accumulate, with a recirculation of stale air. There are also reports that in some aircraft, air from smoking cabins is recirculated to the non-smoking compartment after such treatments as dilution, filtration and electrostatic precipitation.

Given the shrinking world resources of energy, a continuous expend-iture of up to 0.7 kW per smoker is rapidly becoming an unacceptable luxury in any enclosed space. Moreover, even if the fuel could be spared, the majority of citizens (both smokers and non-smokers) are unwilling that they should accept any increase of cost as the price for control of cigarette smoke (Table 8.14).

Voluntary Restrictions

Arguments Pro and Con

The main arguments advanced in favour of voluntary restriction of smoking are that legislation is difficult to enforce, that contempt for the law is created by legislating restrictions, and that many otherwise honest citizens will gain a court record for what is regarded as a minor offence.

An analogy may possibly be drawn to another problem of modern society – inconsiderate parking. In Canada, shopping plazas are generally built on private property, and drivers are thus immune from prosecution in such places unless the owner of the plaza lodges a specific complaint with the police. Voluntary restrictions are thus placed on parking in areas reserved for the disabled and in fire-lanes adjacent to stores. Nevertheless, such regulations are frequently ignored, particularly by those with a compelling urge to buy a package of cigarettes! Indeed, parking restrictions on the highway are also ignored unless reinforced by a heavy fine ($50-$60) and/or impounding of the vehicle.

Success to Date

Voluntary restrictions have had rather limited success in controlling smoking. In one study of a large office (Oasis, 1978), almost a quarter of non-smokers had made informal efforts to stop others from smoking in their work area; 52% of those questioned stated that they had been unsuccessful, while 34% had achieved 'mixed' results. The provision of non-smoking areas in aircraft, trains and buses has legislative backing in some countries, but in many jurisdictions the segregation of passengers remains on a semi-voluntary basis. In the latter circumstance, the non-smoker is frequently annoyed by a heavy cigarette smoker who insists upon 'lighting up' in the prohibited areas. Railway systems commonly have by-laws, with hypothetical fines for those who smoke

Table 9.1: Areas Where a Request Made or Received to Stop Smoking

Location	Non-smoker %	Ex-smoker %	Smoker %
Non-smoking area	27.0	22.6	18.6
Other enclosed space	15.4	17.2	17.9

Source: Based on data from Shephard & LaBarre, 1976.

in non-smoking compartments. In Toronto, such rules are usually observed during business hours, when the trains are heavily travelled. However, the same rules are frequently ignored during the evenings; both alcohol ingestion and lesser proximity of other passengers probably contribute to this change of behaviour. One form of voluntary segregation that has worked fairly well (at some cost to operators) has been the assignment of smokers to separate rooms in restaurants and hotels. Nevertheless, the number of restaurant proprietors who are willing to make such arrangements on a voluntary basis has been quite small.

The frequency of violation of non-smoking areas is indicated by the fact that, in Toronto, 27% of non-smokers had asked someone to stop smoking within a designated area, and 19% of smokers admitted receiving such a request (Shephard & LaBarre, 1977). Moreoever, 6% of smokers felt it was unreasonable to be asked politely not to smoke even within a non-smoking area (Table 9.1), and 12.6% thought it was unreasonable that such a request should be made in a confined space not specifically designated as a non-smoking area.

Extension of Restrictions

Despite violations of existing restrictions, the majority of smokers were either indifferent to or in favour of the establishment of more non-smoking areas in public facilities. The usual reason stated for advocating such a development was a wish to give up smoking in order to conserve future health (Table 9.1). Continued health education would thus seem important not only as a means of curing the cigarette addict, but also as a factor in extending the protection of the non-smoker against passive accumulations of cigarette smoke.

Legislation

A Counsel of Despair

Over the present century, the habit of cigarette smoking has become so pervasive in Western society that with a few exceptions, such as temples and church sanctuaries, the smoker has assumed an implicit right to indulge his or her habit.

This assumption has naturally been fostered by the powerful vested interests of tobacco manufacturing and, until recently, many authors believed that the prospect of enacting effective control legislation was negligible (Fisher, 1962; Maxwell, 1962; James, 1964; Long, 1964). In 1963, Neuberger noted that the Library of Congress contained 30 legislative proposals intended to deal with various aspects of the smoking problem. Not one of these proposals had been accorded even a perfunctory hearing in Congress, all being dismissed at the committee stage.

Only ten years ago, many of the courts also favoured the smoker. For instance, a German taxi-driver was fined 50 DM for having the audacity to tell a passenger rather bluntly not to smoke inside his vehicle (Eberle, 1977).

The Changing Tide of Public Opinion

In the United Kingdom, opinions began to change with the report of the Royal College of Physicians on Smoking and Health (1962). Among other measures to curb the rising consumption of tobacco, the College suggested a much wider restriction of smoking in public places.

Opinions in the US were strongly influenced by a series of well-documented reports on Smoking and Health from the Surgeon General. Legislation restricting smoking in public places has now been proposed in 45 of the 50 US states, exceptions being jurisdictions where tobacco growing makes a major contribution to the economy (Vanderslice, 1976). Unfortunately, less than half of the states have yet enacted these legislative proposals (National Clearing House, 1976, 1977; Center for Disease Control, 1978). However, several large cities such as New York and Chicago have adopted comprehensive municipal regulations restricting smoking in public places.

A turning point for European countries was the recommendation of the Council of Europe (1973) that smoking should be prohibited in all enclosed public facilities, particularly means of transport. In Germany, a dentist brought a successful action against the Schleswig-Holstein Dental Association for unwilling exposure to cigarette smoke at a legally-required continuing education course (Medizinische Monatschrift, 1975). A civil court ruled that in such a situation, the appellant was entitled to freedom from harm or inconvenience unrelated to the prime purpose of the event. One factor in reaching judgement against the Dental Association was the argument that adverse health effects from the passive smoke exposure could not be *excluded*. In 1974, only three years after the unfortunate non-smoking taxi-driver had been fined, a similar dispute arose in a West German taxi-cab. However, on this occasion the court ruled in favour of the non-smoking vehicle operator (Eberle, 1977). A key factor in the revised decision was the view that on current evidence, the driver's health *could* have been endangered by the passenger's cigarettes.

Current Situation

Many nations have now enacted legislation at federal, provincial or municipal levels restricting or prohibiting smoking in public places. Examples include: Austria, Belgium, Bulgaria, Canada, Denmark, East Germany, Finland, France, Italy, Poland, Singapore, South Africa, Sweden, United Kingdom, USA, USSR and West Germany (WHO, 1976; Schwartz, 1977; South African Dept. of Health, 1977; Tobacco, 1977; Vosburgh & Vosburgh, 1977; L'Heureux, 1979). Specific targets of such legislation have included elevators, trains, taxi-cabs, theatres, museums, concert halls, shops and lecture halls.

It seems worth comment that two countries resistant to the introduction of such laws (Greece and Turkey) both have state-controlled tobacco monopolies (WHO, 1976). It is also suggested that the British government has been hesitant to adopt more stringent control legislation because many tobacco manufacturers have their head offices within the UK (L'Heureux, 1979).

Government Buildings

The US government now severely restricts smoking in buildings that fall under its control. Designated non-smoking areas include auditoriums, elevators and shuttle vehicles. Smoking is allowed in conference rooms only if ventilation is adequate, or air-cleaning equipment is installed. Cafeterias, working areas and medical care facilities must provide separate and clearly signed areas for smokers and non-smokers. Government employees may also request a smoke-free work area, provided that this does not require costly additions or alterations to the workplace, and the efficiency of working teams remains unimpaired (Federal Register, 1976, 1979).

Aircraft

The US Civil Aeronautics Board ruled in 1973 that 'certificated' air carriers must provide designated non-smoking areas on all of their aircraft. Further, it was required that the number of seats allocated be sufficient to accommodate all passengers requiring non-smoking accommodation, and carriers were responsible for taking all necessary action to enforce these regulations. When the legislation was first introduced, it was opposed by most carriers, on the grounds that trade would be lost to airlines that permitted smoking. However, history has shown that the carriers of most other nations have found it necessary to follow the US lead in this matter. Initially, 15% of seats were reserved for non-smokers, but this allocation has grown rapidly to 60–70%, encouraged by consumer demand and a fine of $10,000 levied against Eastern Airlines for their failure to provide requested non-smoking accommodation. In general, separation of the two categories of passenger has cut down friction between smokers and non-smokers. Nevertheless, in 1980, the US Civil Aeronautics Board still received 708 complaints concerning smoking violations (3% of all complaints) and $3,500 in fines were levied against US carriers. Furthermore, the need to segregate smokers inevitably slows down the issuing of boarding passes, and may leave aircraft with unused seating capacity. A complete ban upon smoking has thus been proposed for short-haul aircraft. Proponents of the revised policy argue that the public will now watch a film for two hours without smoking, and a similar period of abstinence should be possible on board an aircraft. Moreover, the USSR has found it possible to prohibit smoking on all flights of less than five hours duration. Such action is particularly welcome on commuter services, where small cabins preclude effective separation of smokers from non-smokers. Total prohibition of smoking on inter-continental flights is a more debatable issue — passengers with a strong addiction to cigarettes might then adopt the annoying and dangerous expedient of smoking in the aircraft washrooms.

Hospitals and Doctors' Offices

Perhaps the most logical place to begin the enforcement of a clean-air policy is in health facilities. However, progress in this area has been disappointing. A study of US Physicians (Medical Tribune, 1978) established that only 22% were current smokers. Some 84% of doctors indicated that they encouraged smoking withdrawal, yet only 58% actually prohibited smoking inside their offices and waiting rooms. The Canadian Hospital Association passed a resolution in 1975 asking all hospitals to prohibit smoking in areas used specifically for patient care; institutions were also asked to create smoke-free zones in more generally used areas such as waiting rooms and cafeterias (Campbell,

1976). A subsequent survey showed that only 66% of respondent hospitals had any smoking policy (67% of larger and 58% of smaller hospitals). Smoking was prohibited in 85-90% of heart and chest wards, 47% of psychiatric wards, 45% of maternity wards, 37% of general wards and 60% of out-patient departments. In 63% of institutions, enforcement was the responsibility of the doctor and/or nurse, and in 25% the fire marshal was responsible. Fifty-six per cent of respondents admitted that the regulations were only partially enforced. In January 1977, the Provincial Health Minister 'invited' Québecois hospitals to identify separate 'sectors' for smokers and non-smokers; he further expressed a hope that certain 'more audacious' administrators might prohibit the use of tobacco on hospital premises (L'Heureux, 1979); however, to date there has been no analysis of responses to this invitation.

In Britain, the restriction of smoking in hospitals formed part of an anti-smoking drive that was begun in 1977 (Tobacco, 1977). Among Scottish hospitals, regulations were more commonly directed against the smoking of visitors (67%) than that of nurses (44%) or patients (12%) (Crofton, *et al.*, 1977).

The American Cancer Society began a campaign in 1973 against the sale of cigarettes in hospitals (Dowdell, 1973/4). At this time, 78% of hospitals in Connecticutt had written smoking policies, 71% prohibiting the sale of tobacco products, 71% regulating smoking by visitors and 37% banning employees from smoking while at duty stations (Davis, 1975). By 1976, only 43% of respondent hospitals in Metropolitan Washington DC consistently agreed to requests by patients for non-smoking rooms, eleven of 21 hospitals still sold cigarettes, and four out of 21 permitted staff to smoke within the patients' rooms (Fishman, 1976).

Schools

Another priority area for clean-air legislation is the schoolroom. In 1977, the Quebec Minister of Education called upon all provincial school boards to define areas where smoking was prohibited, and even to stop all smoking within schools (L'Heureux, 1979). Particularly progressive policies have been adopted by the State of Oregon (Oregon State Board of Education, 1972). Directives to local school boards recognize that schools were not designed to accommodate a large number of smokers, and that health, safety, educational responsibilities and the rights of the non-smoker must all weigh heavily against the claims of older students who wish to smoke. Michigan, also, prohibits smoking inside school buildings (Michigan State Dept. of Education, 1971). However, smoking in defiance of regulations remains a major disciplinary problem (Brody, 1977). Enforcement of the rule makes heavy demands upon faculty time, and creates an attitude of rebellion that encourages some students to smoke. One expedient has been to establish outdoor areas where students over the age of 18 are permitted to smoke.

Compliance and Enforcement

A major concern with all legislation is compliance. In theory, Finland has now enacted very strong legislation, which prohibits smoking in all public places; nevertheless, one newspaper report from Helsinki suggested that 'ash-trays were still in banks and customers were still smoking as usual'. Equally, the only penalty imposed upon those who smoke in Russian restaurants is a refusal of service, and this hazard can too often be avoided by a suitable tipping of the waiter (L'Heureux, 1979).

In Italy, individuals who violate smoking regulations are now liable to fines of 1,000–10,000 lira ($1.25–$12.50), while operators of facilities who do not display appropriate signs are subject to penalties of $25–$125. Interestingly, institutional penalties can be augmented by 50% if the ventilation system is not functioning or is shown to be inadequate.

Legislation enacted by the city of Ottawa introduced maximum fines of $1,000 for smoking offences. Parking control officers were charged with enforcement of the regulations. A similar law was introduced in Toronto, but less satisfactorily the enforcement was left to the operator of the building.

Varying methods of enforcement have been adopted by US cities and states. In New York, penalties for violation of anti-smoking laws can theoretically reach $1,000, with one year of imprisonment in the event of non-payment. However, a typical convicted offender pays from $10–$25. Chicago now boasts a special 'smokers' court', and this is exacting fines of $50 to $300 from up to 800 violators per year (Vosburgh & Vosburgh, 1977; L'Heureux, 1979). Minnesota prohibits smoking in most public places except bars; people violating the regulations are fined up to $100, and proprietors of establishments who repeatedly fail to make reasonable efforts to enforce the law are subject to court injunctions (Brandt & Matczynski, 1976).

A survey conducted in Berkeley, California, found 70% of residents in favour of the ordinances introduced to date (85% of non-smokers and 34% of smokers). Only 54% of business people expressed approval; nevertheless, most of them had encountered little difficulty in enforcing the regulations, and 92% considered that their level of business had been unaffected. Significant non-compliance with the regulations persists, and 57% of non-smokers had found it necessary to ask someone to stop smoking on at least one occasion since the laws had been introduced (Sanford *et al.*, 1978).

In Minnesota, a recent survey was more encouraging (Gottier, 1979). In general, regulation was apparently effective. Restaurants had allocated their more attractive seating areas to non-smokers. Hospitals were complying with the law in treatment areas, but less completely in areas occupied by the general public and staff. Large departmental and grocery stores were also enforcing the law, although the situation was less satisfactory with respect to smaller businesses such as barbers' shops. The Health Department was receiving about 100 reports of non-compliance per month, and in 85% of instances the party cited had proved co-operative in remedying the situation. The police were issuing citations, where necessary, for violation of the regulations.

An alternative basis to enforcement is the monitoring of airborne particulate matter (Sem & Tsurubayashi, 1975). Japanese authorities have set the maximum allowable concentration of particles less than 10μ in size at $150 \mu g \cdot m^3$ for buildings with a floor area of more than $3,000 m^2$. The statute covers departmental stores, offices, apartment buildings and public buildings. Table 3.3 suggests that the proposed standard provides good protection against the accumulation of cigarette smoke.

Constitutional Validity

The constitutional validity of legislation continues to be the subject of much discussion. The main bases for legal action have been: (i) health hazards; (ii) public nuisance; and (iii) fire hazards (Pollard & Brennan, 1978).

In one recent court hearing, a non-smoker who complained of exposure to cigarette smoke at the Louisiana Superdome stadium lost his case; the judge ruled that the patron had voluntarily decided to attend the stadium, and that therefore he had no constitutional right to 'privacy' (which would include unpolluted air) (Pollard & Brennan, 1978). A civil action involving smoke exposure at work, on the other hand, was settled in favour of the non-smoker. Two important differences were noted by the judge who conducted the latter hearing: (i) the appellant was obliged to remain within the polluted area during normal working hours; and (ii) there was specific medical evidence of an allergy to the cigarette smoke whereas medical and aesthetic complaints in the Superdome case were only general in nature (Shimp *et al.*, 1976). Nevertheless, not all industrial cases have been decided in favour of non-smokers. In Baden-Wuerttemberg, a construction engineer recently sued his employer, demanding the opportunity to work in a smoke-free room (Medizinische-Welt, 1978). The Labour Tribunal reviewed three possibilities for a favourable settlement of the grievance (prohibition of smoking within the office, a mandatory upgrading of ventilation or allocation of the requested smoke-free room). It decided it did not have authority to prohibit smoking within the office area, added ventilation was rejected as too costly (and possibly annoying to other workers) and a separate room was ruled undesirable because of separation of the employee from his supervisor. The tribunal ruled there was no categoric proof of adverse health effects from passive smoking, and the case was thus dismissed.

Relief is sometimes sought on the basis of the individual's right to 'physical integrity' (L'Heureux, 1979). Nevertheless, it is widely accepted that passive smoking cannot be controlled completely by law. The remedy is rather a general change of societal attitudes (Boex, 1972).

In Canada, there has been much discussion of a possible basis for legal action, but a federal statute has yet to be enacted to give relief to non-smokers. Federal law accepts the concept of a 'criminal public nuisance', but a conviction on such grounds would require clear proof of danger to life, safety or public health, or alternatively good evidence that physical injury had been caused to the individual (L'Heureux, 1979). Under Provincial Labour laws, an employee in Ontario can refuse to work if he believes his health to be in imminent danger; unfortunately, it has been ruled that the danger presented by dense cigarette smoke is not an 'imminent' danger to health, and this is therefore not a ground for ceasing work. On the other hand, the Province has undertaken a campaign to establish (in full consultation with the workers), smoke-free zones in office buildings under its control. Recent municipally enacted legislation has already faced court challenges. In food stores, a health hazard can be argued, and this is properly a municipal concern. In other types of building, the concern is related to air pollution, and it could be argued that this falls under provincial rather than municipal jurisdiction. The Province of Ontario recently reviewed municipal by-laws, and concluded that prohibitions of smoking were legal, provided that the onus for enforcement was placed upon an inspecting agency rather than the proprietor. Nevertheless, the Province has recommended that legislation be introduced only where public co-operation and compliance may be anticipated (Ontario Ministry of Health, 1976). Self-regulatory guidelines are proposed for such areas as transportation, restaurants, health facilities and educational institutions. The Provincial document suggests that the prospects for acceptance of the guidelines will be increased through: (i) promotion of smoke-free zones by government, health organizations and citizen activity; (ii) public demand for smoke-free areas; (iii) encouragement of managements to modify buildings and operations to create a smoke-free environment; (iv) willingness of management to provide the necessary supervision; and (v) co-operation of the general public.

To date, the Tobacco Manufacturers' Council has maintained a relatively low profile in all of this controversy. However, it has sponsored a series of advertisements stressing the considerate nature of most smokers, and pleading for a matching 'reasonableness' on the part of non-smokers. Official pronouncements from the manufacturers' research laboratories have maintained that investigators demonstrating adverse effects have used unrealistically high smoke concentrations (US House of Representatives, 1978), that the supposed health hazards from both active and passive smoking are poorly documented, that freedom of choice must be conserved and that tobacco farming makes an important contribution to the US economy (Dwyer, 1978).

10 PASSIVE SMOKING AND THE FETUS

The fetus is in a unique and unfortunate situation, since many of the toxic gases and vapours inhaled by the mother are transported to it via the placental circulation. It is at special risk if the mother smokes during pregnancy. A combination of local oxygen want and rapidly differentiating tissues set the threshold of tobacco smoke toxicity far below the standards accepted for an adult. Maternal smoking thus invokes a sad litany of problems including prematurity, low birth weight, increased perinatal mortality and an impairment of development that continues throughout much of childhood. Problems may be compounded further by a secretion of toxic chemicals into maternal milk. The present chapter will assess the magnitude of such risks, and will assess attitudes towards smoking during pregnancy and the puerperium.

Smoking Patterns of Women

It has been suspected for many years that both nicotine exposure and cigarette smoke have an adverse effect upon the development of the fetus (Ballantyne, 1902; Guillan & Gy, 1907; Fleig, 1908). Animal experiments have given clear evidence that exposure to smoke constituents causes both a low birth weight and an increased proportion of stillbirths (Sodano, 1934; Pechstein & Reynolds, 1937; Essenberg *et al.*, 1940; Schoeneck, 1941; Willson, 1942).

However, it was not until World War II that an epidemic of smoking by women made this phenomenon a major public health problem. Statistics for the US illustrate the point. During and immediately following World War II, some 37% of the cohort of women born in 1911–20 were regular cigarette smokers, and by 1960 some 45% of the 1921–30 and 1931–40 cohorts had also become regular smokers (US Surgeon General, 1980). Since the mid-1960s, the proportion of smokers has declined in all birth cohorts, and there has been an increased usage of low-tar, low nicotine filter-tip cigarettes. On the other hand, there has been a dramatic increase in the daily cigarette consumption by those women who continue to smoke. Thus, in 1965, 44.5% of US female smokers consumed less than 15 cigarettes per day, and only

13.7% consumed more than 25 cigarettes per day. However, by 1979 the corresponding figures were 34.6% and 22.4% (US Surgeon General, 1980). Approximately a third of continuing smokers make a serious attempt to quit smoking in any given year, but only about one in five of these succeed in their attempt.

Currently, about 35% of North American women of child-bearing age are smokers (US Surgeon General, 1980). About 80% of female smokers who become pregnant claim some reduction of their cigarette consumption during pregnancy; many suggest a 50% decrease in cigarette usage and about a quarter stop smoking entirely (Langford *et al.*, 1980). However, the immediate response rate remains uninfluenced by educational programmes, and it is improbable that the habits of many women change in the critical early weeks of pregnancy, before antenatal education has begun.

Possible Mechanisms

A variety of mechanisms have been suggested whereby maternal smoking habits could influence fetal health; these include the underlying constitution of the smoker, changes of nutrition and impaired oxygen delivery, as well as more specific effects of nicotine and polycyclic aromatic hydrocarbons upon the parents, the uterus and the fetus (Royal College of Physicians, 1977; Pirani, 1978; US Surgeon General, 1979, 1980).

Constitution

Since the habit of smoking is not randomly assigned to 50% of mothers, it is difficult to refute the hypothesis that smokers are an abnormal group, with complications of pregnancy and the puerperium arising from this abnormality rather than from the contamination of placental blood with tobacco smoke constituents.

Yerushalmy (1965, 1972) is a strong exponent of this view. He has advanced statistics showing that future smokers have a high proportion of low birth weight infants *before* they start smoking, and that former smokers conceive an unusually high percentage of twins. However, there are now several reports which show that the adverse effects of smoking are avoided if a woman stops smoking during the first four months of pregnancy (Schwartz *et al.*, 1972; Naeye, 1978b; Rantakallio, 1978a). Perhaps the most convincing answer to Yerushalmy is the study of Naeye (1978b), where women smoked in one pregnancy, but not in a second. Despite this crossover control of constitutional variables, the influence of smoking upon birth weight persisted.

Nutrition

It is widely accepted that cigarette smoking tends to reduce nutrient intake, whether it acts directly upon the satiety centres, increases the blood sugar, damages the senses of taste and smell or operates less directly through psychological mechanisms (Rode *et al.*, 1972). Some authors have thus suggested that a low birth weight might arise from impairment of maternal appetite and a low maternal weight gain (Davies *et al.*, 1976; Rush, 1979). Animal experiments have shown a decrease of both DNA and total protein in fetuses taken from smoke-exposed mothers (Haworth & Ford, 1972). The data suggest a normal cell size, but either a slowing of cell proliferation or an acceleration of cell breakdown.

The nutritional hypothesis is seductive for a dedicated smoker. It seems much easier to eat a little more than to curtail smoking (Lancet, 1979). The influence of length of gestation, and the impact of the weight of the infant upon maternal weight gain inevitably lead to a certain correlation between birth weight and the increase in weight of the mother. Nevertheless, several recent studies have failed to confirm the overall nutritional hypothesis. The effect of smoking upon birth weight is still seen if women are compared on a basis of equal maternal weight gain, and moreover, in the US at least, the mean gain of smoking mothers during pregnancy exceeds the National Research Council recommendation (Miller & Hassanein, 1964).

After analysing data from 31,788 births in Ontario, Meyer (1978) concluded that maternal smoking was associated with a low birth weight, but was unrelated to the weight gain of the mother. Several recent studies have reached similar conclusions (Jarvinen & Osterlund, 1963; Miller & Hassanein, 1964; Mau & Netter, 1974; Persson *et al.*, 1978). Hajeri *et al.* (1979) matched smokers and non-smokers with respect to age, height, weight at conception, parity and length of gestation. The source of weight gain was also analysed carefully. It was found that the mean extrauterine weight gain during pregnancy averaged 7.04 kg for smokers and 6.90 kg for non-smokers. The conclusion that is reached still depends upon the skill with which intervening variables are controlled. Maternal weight gain tends to increase with the length of gestation, and is lower for a second than a first pregnancy (Naeye, 1978b). Furthermore, birth weight is strongly correlated with maternal size, so that a heavy woman who smokes may give the

misleading appearance of escaping the general cigarette-induced retardation of fetal growth (Garn *et al.*, 1977).

Although the general hypothesis of nutritional impairment is now
discredited, there remain occasional reports that smoking influences
the intake of specific nutrients. Crosby *et al.* (1977) noted low blood
levels of carotene and 14 amino acids in smoking mothers; moreover,
the observed differences from non-smokers (10–20%) were judged
sufficiently large to slow fetal growth. Likewise, Wingerd & Sponzilli
(1977) found low serum globulin values in smokers.

McGarry & Andrews (1972) reported a deficiency of vitamin B_{12}
among smoking mothers. This persisted after adjustment for interfering
variables such as parity and social class. It was attributed to cyanide
detoxification, cyanide being a significant constituent of cigarette
smoke. Schorah *et al.* (1978) described a deficiency of ascorbic acid
in the leucocytes of smokers. The effect was proportional to cigarette
consumption. Schorah *et al.* (1978) argued that lack of vitamin C might
limit fetal development, and predispose to premature rupture of the
amniotic membranes. On the other hand, Yeung (1976) found no
difference in plasma levels of vitamins A, C or E between smokers and
non-smokers. Presumably, where differences have been described,
these could arise in part from socio-economic differences between
smokers and non-smokers. Furthermore, if a non-smoker is a health-
conscious individual, she is more likely to ingest additional protein
and vitamins during pregnancy.

Animal studies suggest that nicotine inhibits lactation (Hatcher &
Crosby, 1927; Thienes *et al.*, 1946; Blake & Sawyer, 1972). Smoking
could thus impair nutrition of the child during the puerperium, if not
during pregnancy.

Oxygen Delivery

Oxygen delivery to the fetus is marginal for survival during the final
three months of pregnancy. The act of smoking erodes the precarious
margin of safety, worsening the respiratory status of the fetus through:
(i) increases in blood levels of carbon monoxide and carbon dioxide;
(ii) decreases of blood oxygen tension; (iii) changes in blood flow
patterns; (iv) inhibition of respiratory enzymes; and (v) placental
complications (particularly bleeding before delivery).

The blocking of both maternal and fetal haemoglobin by carbon
monoxide places the fetus at risk of serious oxygen want during both
the final weeks of growth and the delivery process. Chemical structures
are such that fetal haemoglobin has a much stronger affinity for carbon

monoxide than does maternal haemoglobin. Maternal smoking thus leads to a selective accumulation of carbon monoxide in fetal blood. Transfer of carbon monoxide across the human placenta has a half-time of 1½–2 hours. With an acute exposure to carbon monoxide, the blood COHb of the fetus lags behind that of the mother. Maternal readings are not approached for 5–6 hours, and 36–48 hours may be required for full equilibration. However, the final fetal blood carboxyhaemoglobin level is 10–15% above that of the mother (Longo, 1970, 1977; Hill *et al.*, 1977). Normal patterns of smoking yield relatively stable fetal carboxyhaemoglobin levels, although there is some decrease of COHb at night and in the early morning. Most measurements have been made on umbilical cord blood at the time of delivery. It is likely that in such circumstances, smoking is considerably less than in the remainder of pregnancy. Nevertheless, typical values are 0.2–3.6% in the offspring of non-smokers, compared with 1.1–9.2% in children born to smokers (Heron, 1962).

Carbon monoxide exposure has little influence on arterial oxygen pressure in the adult smoker; however, it leads to a decrease of fetal arterial oxygen pressure (Longo & Hill, 1977). For example, if the fetal blood carboxyhaemoglobin rises to 10%, the arterial oxygen pressure drops from a normal value of 20 torr down to a hypoxic 15.5 torr, while the venous tension drops from 16 to 12.5 torr. A shift of the oxygen dissociation curve also hampers release of oxygen from haemoglobin within the tissue capillaries (Longo, 1972).

The adult subject compensates for carbon monoxide poisoning by an increase of cardiac output, with a corresponding increase in the blood flow to the vital organs (Ayres *et al.*, 1970). However, the fetal heart is already operating near to its maximal capacity, even in the absence of carbon monoxide (Power & Longo, 1975), so that there is little possibility of increasing cardiac output. The main basis of compensation for the decreased oxygen delivery within the fetus is thus a compensatory redirection of the circulation towards the brain, heart and adrenal glands (Longo *et al.*, 1978; US Surgeon General, 1979, 1980).

The mother also attempts to compensate for the poor oxygen delivery to her child, developing a larger and thinner placenta than that found in a non-smoker (Longo, 1972). However, a large, thin placenta is a mixed blessing for the fetus, since it increases the risk of birth complications such as placenta praevia (Christianson, 1979). Immediately following birth, the children of smoking mothers show a metabolic acidosis; this persists for up to 12 hours (Younoszai *et al.*, 1968).

Davies et al. (1976) calculated that if a woman stopped smoking during pregnancy, a combination of a normalization of the oxygen dissociation curve and a reduction of blood carboxyhaemoglobin, increased the oxygen available to the fetus by 8%.

The acute effects of carbon monoxide exposure can have a disastrous effect upon the unborn child. In one series of animal experiments, Longo & Hill (1977) observed that 57% of fetuses sustaining a blood carboxyhaemoglobin level of 15% for 30 minutes subsequently died. Ginsberg & Myers (1976) exposed pregnant monkeys to 0.1–0.3% carbon monoxide, and found that as a result the oxygen content of fetal blood dropped from 9–15 ml/100 ml to less than 2 ml/100 ml. Associated changes included a slowing of the heart, acidosis, a build-up of carbon dioxide, a fall of blood pressure and electrocardiographic evidence of myocardial oxygen lack. In humans, fetal breathing movements are depressed or even arrested for up to 90 minutes after the mother has been smoking (Gennser et al., 1975; Manning & Feyerabend, 1976).

Animal experiments indicate that chronic exposure to carbon monoxide during pregnancy decreases birth weight and increases perinatal mortality (Åstrup et al., 1972; Fechter & Annau, 1977). There are also long-term effects upon visual evoked potentials (Dyer et al., 1979), voluntary activity (Garvey & Longo, 1978) and tissue biochemistry (Garvey & Longo, 1978; Newby et al., 1978).

Nicotine

Blood levels of nicotine in pregnant women smokers commonly range from 14 to 41 ng·ml^{-1} (Gennser et al., 1975; Manning & Feyerabend, 1976). Nicotine traverses the placental barrier quite rapidly (Hansson & Schmiterlow, 1962; Larson & Silvette, 1969); in mice, concentrations within the fetus remain lower than in the mother (Tjalve et al., 1968), but in the rat plasma nicotine concentrations are actually higher in fetal than in maternal blood (Mosier & Jansons, 1973). The drug is apparently distributed preferentially to the adrenal glands, heart and kidneys of the fetus, because of the circulatory changes noted above. Clearance by the liver is slower than in the mother (Tjalve et al., 1968).

The effects produced upon the mature fetus include a rise of systemic blood pressure, either a directly induced rise or a reflex slowing of heart rate (Sontag & Wallace, 1935), acidosis, hypoxia and changes in the excitability of the central nervous system (Sontag & Wallace, 1935; Martin & Becker, 1971; Suzuki et al., 1971; Hudson et al., 1973). The neural disturbances reflect a slowing in the development of neural excitatory and inhibitory pathways, and thus persist after delivery (Martin & Becker, 1971).

In addition to direct pharmacological effects, nicotine increases maternal epinephrine, norepinephrine and cortisol concentrations, causing short-term decreases in blood flow to the uterus and placenta (Armitage, 1965; Haberman-Brueschke *et al.*, 1965; Lehtovirta & Forss, 1978; Quigley *et al.*, 1979; Resnik *et al.*, 1979). It may also cause a vasoconstriction of the uterine blood vesicles, with a decrease in the perfusion of the inter-villous spaces (Suzuki *et al.*, 1971). Finally an increase of red cell size raises blood viscosity, further restricting blood flow to both maternal and fetal sides of the placenta (Harrison & McKenna, 1977).

Within the placenta, nicotine depresses cellular metabolism, thus blocking active transport of amino acids from the maternal to the fetal circulation (Tanaka, 1965); this could have serious implications for fetal growth (Rowel & Sastry, 1977, 1978). There have also been reports of abnormal vascular morphology in the placentae of smokers (Loehr *et al.*, 1972; Asmussen & Kjeldsen, 1975; Asmussen, 1977; Spira *et al.*, 1977). Other acute effects of nicotine upon the mother include an increase of oxygen consumption, hypoglycaemia and an increased usage of fatty acids (Abel, 1980).

Chronic experiments on various animal models suggest that implantation of the ovum is delayed by smoking. Nicotine disturbs the normal balance of sex hormones, leading to a decrease of progesterone, luteinizing hormone and prolactin, with above normal concentrations of oestrogen and follicle stimulating hormones (Yoshinaga *et al.*, 1979). Regular dosage with nicotine ($1 \text{ mg} \cdot \text{kg}^{-1} \text{ day}^{-1}$) results in a decreased litter size, and an increased stillbirth rate (Hamosh *et al.*, 1979), with slow growth after birth due to a poor maternal milk secretion (Hatcher & Crosby, 1927; Thienes *et al.*, 1946; Hamosh *et al.*, 1979). Similar effects upon milk output have been described in women who smoke (Thompson, 1933; but not Underwood *et al.*, 1965). Unfortunately, it is difficult to disentangle the influence of personality, since anxiety and smoking are commonly associated. Anxiety rather than cigarettes may therefore be responsible for any problems of lactation.

Nicotine is readily secreted by the human breast ducts (Hatcher & Crosby, 1927; Thompson, 1933; Perlman *et al.*, 1942), and can be detected in milk up to eight hours after smoking (Emanuel, 1931). Emanuel (1931) reported a maximum concentration of only 0.03 $\text{mg} \cdot \text{l}^{-1}$ but others have observed values ranging from 0.12 $\text{mg} \cdot \text{l}^{-1}$ for a light smoker to 0.5 $\text{mg} \cdot \text{l}^{-1}$ in an individual smoking 11–20 cigarettes per day (Perlman *et al.*, 1942). Discrepancies may relate to the method of sampling. Emanuel tested wet nurses, while other authors examined the residual milk after nursing had been completed. Early analyses were also based upon ingenious but unreliable bioassays, using such organisms as leeches and daphnia. Ferguson *et al.* (1976) developed a more satisfactory gas chromatographic method of analysis; using this procedure, milk nicotine concentrations of 20 to 512 ppb (approximately 0.02–0.51 mg·l^{-1}) were found. Such figures suggest that heavy smokers provide their babies at each feeding with as much nicotine per unit of body weight as they themselves obtain from a single cigarette. There are occasional anecdotal reports of 'nicotine poisoning' among infants whose mothers were heavy smokers (Greiner, 1936; Bisdom, 1937).

Polycyclic Aromatic Hydrocarbons

Polycyclic aromatic hydrocarbons such as benzo (α) pyrene are a major concern in view of their known mutagenic and carcinogenic properties. The possibility of harming the unborn child here extends to the male partner, since smoking increases the number of chromosomal aberrations in both male and female germ cells (Viczian, 1969; Obe & Herha, 1978; Lambert *et al.*, 1978). Although the mutagenic effect is relatively weak, there are sufficient smokers in most populations to have a significant impact upon the total genetic pool (Bridges *et al.*, 1979).

Placental transfer of benzo (α) pyrene has been studied in terms of the increased activity of the enzyme aryl hydrocarbon hydroxylase. Since the dose of benzo (α) pyrene needed to induce such an effect was greater in the fetus than in the adult, Welch *et al.* (1972) argued that the placenta offered some protection against this compound. However, an alternative explanation of their findings is that the enzyme system of the fetus was immature, and thus less readily induced. In any event, there is good evidence that some benzo (α) pyrene penetrates to the fetal circulation (Schlede & Merker, 1972), and in animals at least the offspring show a correspondingly increased risk of neoplasms of the lungs, liver and mammary glands (Bulay & Wattenberg, 1970; Nikonova, 1977). One study of humans showed a 30% greater incidence of tumours in the children of smokers, but unfortunately the sample size was insufficient to establish the significance of this trend (Neutel & Buck, 1971). The ability of benzo (α) pyrene to induce various enzyme systems blocks a number of active transport processes in the placenta (Welch *et al.*, 1968; Juchau, 1971), thus interfering with fetal nutrition.

Other Smoke Constituents

Relatively little is yet known about the impact of other smoke constituents upon pregnancy and infant health. Cyanide may help to control maternal hypertension, but it also leads to an increased perinatal mortality, with poor subsequent infant growth (Andrews, 1973). Heavy metals such as cadmium are concentrated in the placenta, and blood concentrations are thus lower in the fetus than in the mother (Lauwerys *et al.*, 1978).

Animal experiments have shown an increase of tumours in the young when their mothers are given nitrosamines (Mohr & Althoff, 1971). This raises the disturbing possibility that the nitrosamines present in cigarette smoke could be transmitted to a baby via its mother's milk. The insecticide content of human milk also increases with the number of cigarettes smoked by the mother (Bradt & Herrenkohl, 1976).

Fetal and Infant Growth

Birth Weight

The birth weight of an infant is a very good overall indicator of prenatal development, and it has a major influence upon perinatal and neonatal mortality rates. For example, if the birth weight is less than 1.5 kg, the neonatal mortality is an alarming 45%. Risks are least for babies weighing 3.5–4.0 kg, and increase again for those weighing more than 4.0 kg (Baird, 1964).

Studies of over 500,000 births have now amply documented that the weight of infants born to mothers who smoke is less than that of children born to non-smokers (Simpson, 1957; US Surgeon General, 1979; Abel, 1980; Table 10.1). The average disadvantage of the smoker's child is about 200 g, and there is about twice the normal risk of bearing an infant that weighs less than 2.5 kg. Body dimensions are all affected. The average length of infants born to smokers is 1.4 cm less than that for the babies of non-smoking mothers (Meredith, 1975), and the head circumference is proportionately smaller (Peterson *et al.*, 1965). A birth weight of less than 2.5 kg is in itself sufficient to cause a thirtyfold increase of neonatal mortality (Chase, 1969). Smoking accounts for at least a third of all low birth weight infants (Meyer *et al.*, 1976; US Surgeon General, 1979); it is a more significant risk factor than maternal height, age, parity, sex of the child, mother's weight before pregnancy, history of previous pregnancies or type of hospital accommodation (public, semi-private or private; Tables 10.2 and 10.3; Lowe, 1959). Further, the adverse effect of smoking is dose-related. The risk of an

Table 10.1: Percentages of Children Weighing Less than 2.5 kg Born to Smokers and Non-smokers

Study	Per cent births < 2.5 kg	
	Smoking mothers	Non-smoking mothers
Cardiff	8.1	4.1
US Collaborative Study		
White subjects	9.5	4.3
Black subjects	17.5	10.7
California (Kaiser Permanente)		
White subjects	6.4	3.5
Black subjects	13.4	6.4
Montreal	11.4	5.2
Ontario Collaborative Study	9.1	4.5

Source: Based on data from Meyer *et al.*, 1976.

Table 10.2: Relative Risk that a Smoking Mother will Bear an Infant of Less than 2.5 kg Birth Weight, Classified by Interfering Variables

Interfering variable	Relative risk of infant < 2.5 kg	
	< 1 pack/day	> 1 pack/day
Public hospital ward	1.6	2.4
Private hospital accommodation	1.8	2.8
Mother's height < 157.5 cm	1.8	2.6
> 172.7 cm	2.2	3.5
Pre-pregnancy weight < 54.5 kg	1.7	2.6
> 61.3 kg	1.5	2.6
Male child	1.7	2.7
Female child	1.6	2.4

Source: Based on data from Meyer *et al.*, 1976.

underweight child is increased 53% for those women consuming less than a pack of cigarettes per day, but 130% in those smoking more than a pack per day (Meyer *et al.*, 1976; Fielding & Yankauer, 1978). Larger babies are also affected, since smoking displaces the distribution curve of birth weights leftward in a relatively uniform fashion (MacMahon *et al.*, 1966; Figure 10.1).

Yerushalmy (1964, 1972) argued that a particular type of woman both smoked and bore small children, since such an association could be demonstrated in women who did not start to smoke until after their child was born. However, this study has been faulted on several counts, including failure to control for a low average age and a high proportion of first births among the 'future smokers' (Silverman, 1977).

Table 10.3: Difference of Body Weight Between Infants Born to
Smoking and Non-smoking Mothers, Classified by Interfering Biological
and Socio-economic Variables

Interfering variable	Disadvantage of smoker's child (g)
Mother's age < 20 years	193
More than four previous pregnancies	286
Previous birth < 2.5 kg	208
Mother's height < 152 cm	201
Mother's pre-pregnancy weight < 45 kg	246
Mother did not graduate from high school	253
Father did not graduate from high school	256
Husband unskilled labourer or service worker	247

Source: Based on data from Van den Berg, 1977.

Figure 10.1: Birth Weights of Children Born to Non-smoking Mothers
and Mothers who Smoked More than One Pack of Cigarettes Per Day

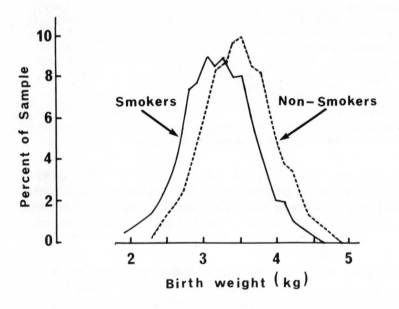

Source: Based on data from MacMahon *et al.*, 1966.

The current concensus is that the growth deficit of the baby is causally related to an impaired supply of oxygen or nutrients, rather than to any constitutional difference in smoking mothers, or a tobacco-induced change of genetic programming (US Surgeon General, 1979). The main evidence for this viewpoint is that a woman who stops smoking early in pregnancy can still bear an infant of normal weight (Lowe, 1959; MacMahon *et al.*, 1966; Schwartz *et al.*, 1972; Silverman, 1977). The critical time for impeding fetal growth is still discussed (Lowe, 1959; Frazier *et al.*, 1961; Herriot *et al.*, 1962; Schwartz *et al.*, 1972; Rantakallio, 1978a), but is likely subsequent to the fourth month of pregnancy (US Surgeon General, 1980). The fact that height remains proportional to weight (Hardy & Mellits, 1972) contrasts with the usual response to maternal malnutrition (a long, thin infant; Miller *et al.*, 1976). Moreover, the small children born to smoking mothers fail to show the 'catch-up' growth that is typical of malnutrition (Miller *et al.*, 1976; Dunn *et al.*, 1976, 1977). We may thus suspect that oxygen lack rather than malnutrition is responsible for the restricted growth.

Placental Development

The placental weight is affected relatively little if the mother smokes (Jarvinen & Osterlund, 1963; O'Lane, 1963; Mulcahy *et al.*, 1970). Given the reduction of fetal weight discussed above, the placental/ fetal ratio is thus increased progressively from 0.171 in a non-smoker to 0.188 in those women consuming more than 20 cigarettes per day (Kullander & Kaellen, 1971; Wilson, 1972; Wingerd *et al.*, 1976). Moreover, the greater relative placental weight seems independent of the duration of gestation, being seen in heavy smokers at all gestational ages from 37 to 43 weeks (Wingerd *et al.*, 1976). According to some recent reports, the placenta of a smoking mother is also thinner than normal, with an increased diameter, more calcification and patchy sub-chorionic fibrin (Christianson, 1979). The greater size is probably an adaptation to hypoxia (Wilson, 1972; Wingerd *et al.*, 1976). Some of the other changes suggest faster aging, possibly an action of smoke constituents upon the placental vessels (Asmussen, 1978).

Length of Gestation

Smoking reduces the duration of gestation by no more than two days (Lowe, 1959; Buncher, 1969; Butler & Alberman, 1969; Bailey, 1970; Kullander & Kaellen, 1971; Andrews & McGarry, 1972; Schwartz *et*

Figure 10.2: Influence of Maternal Smoking Upon Birth Weight, Considered in Relation to the Duration of Gestation

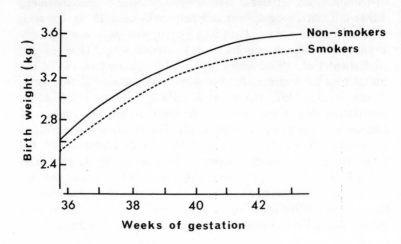

Source: Based on data from Butler and Alberman, 1969.

al., 1972; Yerushalmy, 1972; British Medical Journal, 1978a). The reduction of birth weight thus cannot be explained simply by a shortening of gestation. There is rather a true retardation of intrauterine growth (Persson *et al.*, 1978). The baby that is born is both short and light for dates (Figure 10.2), but is normally proportioned with respect to such dimensions as head and shoulder circumference (Kullander & Kaellen, 1971; Hardy & Mellits, 1972; Davies *et al.*, 1976) and has a normal ponderal index (Miller *et al.*, 1976).

Long-term Growth and Development

The condition of the child immediately after birth is commonly rated in terms of an 'AGPAR score'. Most authors have found such scores to be similar in the children of smokers and non-smokers (Peterson *et al.*, 1965; Russell *et al.*, 1968; Kullander & Kaellen, 1971; Cope *et al.*, 1973; but not O'Lane, 1963). However, there are reports that shortly after birth the children of smokers were less visually alert (Landesman-Dwyer *et al.*, 1978) and performed more poorly than the children of non-smokers on such tasks as head-turning and sucking (Abel, 1980).

Exposure to tobacco constituents during pregnancy apparently has long-lasting effects upon a child's growth and development. At one year, the child of a smoker has a weight deficit of 0.3 kg (Russell *et al.*, 1968; Hardy & Mellits, 1972). This persists throughout childhood. The deficit of stature amounts to 0.9 cm at five years (Wingerd & Schoen, 1974), 1.0 cm (Hardy & Mellits, 1972) or 1.4 cm (Goldstein, 1977) at seven years and 1.6 cm at eleven years of age (Butler & Goldstein, 1973; but not MacMahon *et al.*, 1966). Moreover, it is not possible to account for such differences in terms of other adverse social and biological factors encountered among smoking mothers.

Associated delays of intellectual and emotional development are seen as late as eleven years of age (Hardy & Mellits, 1972; Butler & Goldstein, 1973; Wingerd & Schoen, 1974; Davies *et al.*, 1976; Naeye *et al.*, 1977). Hardy & Mellits (1972) observed that smokers' children have lower average scores on most tests of intelligence and intellectual function at four and seven years of age, even after allowing for such factors as maternal age, education, race, date of delivery and sex of the child. However, because of a relatively small sample size (88 matched pairs), the majority of differences were statistically insignificant. Dunn *et al.* (1976, 1977) reported that minor neurological abnormalities (minimal cerebral dysfunction and abnormal electroencephalograms) were a little more common in the children of women who smoked. Poorer scores were also obtained in 45 of 48 psychological tests, differences being statistically significant in 14 of 48 comparisons. Further, the children of smokers had poorer behaviour ratings and school placements. Analysis of variance established that only a part of these various handicaps could be attributed to interfering socio-economic variables. The most convincing study of postnatal development was based on the 17,000 births that occurred in Great Britain during the period 3-9 March 1958 (Butler & Goldstein, 1973). Data were classified on the basis of the amount smoked per day after the fourth month of pregnancy. After allowing for social factors in the home environment and biological factors including health, 11-year-old children had a persistent 1.5 cm disadvantage of height if their mother had smoked more than ten cigarettes per day; they also had a nine month handicap of reading age and mathematics age (Table 10.4), these differences being highly significant ($P < 0.001$).

Heavy maternal smoking apparently increases the chances that a child will be hyperkinetic (Denson *et al.*, 1975). The average cigarette consumption of mothers with hyperkinetic children is three times that for mothers with normal children. However, this association is not necessarily causal; conceivably, a problem of maternal personality contributed to both the high cigarette consumption and the hyperkinesis.

Table 10.4: Development of 11-year-old Children, Classified According to Smoking Habit of Mother from Fourth Month of Pregnancy

Variable	Cigarette consumption of mother	
	1-9 cigarettes per day	> 10 cigarettes per day
Height retardation (cm)	0.9	1.5
Retardation of reading age (months)	7	9
Retardation of mathematics age (months)	7	9

Source: Based on data from Butler & Goldstein, 1973, adjusted for other social and biological variables.

Saxton (1978) commented on irritability, decreased self-control and a general lack of interest among the children of smoking mothers. He ascribed these problems tentatively to hypoxic damage of the cochlea at a critical stage in their development.

Fetal and Infant Mortality and Morbidity

Abortion

Statistics on the incidence of abortions among smokers are much harder to interpret than effects upon fetal development. A proportion of supposedly 'spontaneous' abortions are self-induced, or procured in backstreet abortion mills, complicating retrospective surveys, while prospective surveys are hampered because smokers enrol in investigations later and less willingly than non-smokers. If only low birth weight infants are considered, the smokers have a lower perinatal mortality than non-smokers. This paradoxical finding arises partly because the small infant of a smoker is more mature than a child of corresponding weight born to a non-smoker (Meyer & Comstock, 1972), and partly because smoking induces a large increase of low birth weight infants but a much smaller increase in the number of abortions.

Despite these various experimental problems, several authors have demonstrated an association between 'spontaneous' abortion and maternal smoking habits (Hudson & Rucker, 1945; Bernhard, 1962; Zabriskie, 1963; Underwood *et al.*, 1965; Russell *et al.*, 1966; Kullander & Kaellen, 1971; Palmgren & Wallander, 1971; Cope *et al.*, 1973; Hollingsworth *et al.*, 1976; Kline *et al.*, 1977; Himmelberger *et al.*, 1978). Even in studies where the increase of fetal and neonatal loss was not statistically significant (Savel & Roth, 1962; O'Lane, 1963; Peterson *et al.*, 1965; Downing & Chapman, 1966; Underwood *et al.*,

1967; Rantakallio, 1969), the mortality ratios for smoking mothers were all greater than unity (1.01 to 1.06). Moreover, the results cannot be ascribed simply to differences of age, marital status, parity or social class (Kline *et al.*, 1977). Nevertheless, it would be rash to attribute the excess of abortions in smoking mothers entirely to a toxic effect of the smoke exposure. Malcolm & Shephard (1978) noted an association between smoking habits and sexual behaviour, and Kullander & Kaellen (1971) pointed out that the excess of abortions among smokers increased from 20% for 'wanted' pregnancies to 35% for 'unwanted' pregnancies. In the latter study, 19% of pregnancies among smokers were unwanted, compared with 13% among non-smokers.

Bearing in mind this problem of interpretation, several studies have set a substantially higher risk of spontaneous abortion for the heavy smoker. Kline *et al.* (1977) calculated an odds ratio of 1:8 for smokers relative to non-smokers. Fergusson (1979) found a doubling of spontaneous abortions among women smoking more than 20 cigarettes per day; moreover, this risk could not be explained by such confounding variables as age, parity, marital status, education or socio-economic status. Likewise, after controlling for other variables, Himmelberger *et al.* (1978) still observed a 70% increase of spontaneous abortions among professional women who smoked.

The proportion of abnormal fetuses aborted is, if anything, lower in a smoker than in a non-smoker. The spontaneous abortions seem to be secondary to other complications of pregnancy rather than to abnormal fetal development (Alberman *et al.*, 1976; British Medical Journal, 1978a).

Congenital Anomalies

Himmelberger *et al.* (1978) found that smoking mothers had an increased risk of bearing live babies with congenital anomalies. This trend persisted after controlling for age, pregnancy history and exposure to anaesthetic gases (Table 10.5). In heavy smokers, the risk was more than doubled. Andrews & McGarry (1972) reported a total of 2.73% abnormal live infants born to smokers, compared with 2.37% for non-smokers; in their series, the largest effect was on the incidence of cleft palate and hare-lip (0.26% versus 0.11%). Fedrick (1978) confirmed this trend and also noted a significant positive association between maternal smoking and congenital heart disease (including persistent ductus arteriosus). Other reported abnormalities include facial development (Mau & Netter, 1974), anencephaly (Naeye, 1979), and various malformations of the central nervous system and special senses

Table 10.5: Percentage of Selected Congenital Abnormalities in Live Babies Born to Smokers and Non-smokers

Type of congenital abnormality	Percentage incidence		Significance of difference[a]
	Smokers	Non-smokers	
Cardiovascular	1.91	1.37	0.02
Urogenital	2.13	1.5?	0.02
Gastro-intestinal	1.35	0 ..	0.04
Musculo-skeletal	2.38	1.97	0.08
Respiratory	1.52	1.21	0.10
Central nervous system	1.15	1.02	0.27

Note: a. One-tailed t-test.
Source: Based on data from Himmelberger *et al.*, 1978.

(Heinonen *et al.*, 1977). However, the increased risk of the smoking mother has typically been quite small, and indeed it has not been confirmed by all investigators. For instance, Borlee & Lechat (1979) found no difference of smoking habits between mothers with normal infants and those whose children were malformed. They pointed out that congenital malformations were associated with a heavy maternal coffee consumption (more than eight cups per day), and suggested that this could lead to an indirect association between smoking and malformation.

Perinatal Mortality

Perinatal mortality refers to deaths of the fetus after 28 weeks of gestation, and of infants aged less than seven days (or in some reports less than 28 days). Analysis of the effects of smoking is complicated, since women with a generally increased risk of perinatal mortality (the very young, the very old, black subjects and those with limited education or a low socio-economic status) are particularly susceptible to the adverse effects of smoking. According to Meyer *et al.* (1975), the risk for light smokers who are young, of low parity and with a normal haemoglobin level is less than 10%. At the other end of the scale, there is a 70–100% increase of risk among anaemic women admitted to public hospital wards with a history of many previous pregnancies including some infants with low birth weights. Using a multiple regression approach to allow for the influence of intervening variables, Meyer *et al.* (1976) established perinatal mortality rates (per 1,000 live births) of 23.5 for non-smokers, 28.2 for women smoking less than one pack of cigarettes per day and 31.8 for women smoking more than one pack per day.

'Low' birth weight infants (< 2.5 kg) born to smoking mothers have a higher average weight and greater overall maturity than 'low' birth weight infants born to non-smokers, and this sometimes masks the effects of smoking (Goldstein, 1977). Nevertheless, most studies have shown an excess of both stillbirths and overall perinatal mortality when the mother smokes (Frazier *et al.*, 1961; Peterson, 1965; Ravenholt *et al.*, 1966; Comstock & Lundin, 1967; Butler & Alberman, 1969; Kullander & Kaellen, 1971; Hardy & Mellits, 1972; Schwartz *et al.*, 1972; Cope *et al.*, 1973; Fabia, 1973; Rush, 1974; Meyer *et al.*, 1976; Rantakallio, 1978a).

The excess of perinatal deaths apparently has no general cause. Stillbirths sometimes reflect antepartum haemorrhage and/or premature separation of the placenta (abruptio placentae), the relative incidence being 0.11% for non-smokers and 0.39% for smokers (Andrews & McGarry, 1972). More commonly, stillbirths are ascribed to 'unknown causes' (Andrews & McGarry, 1972; Goujard *et al.*, 1975). Neonatal deaths (occurring within 28 days of birth) arise from prematurity and related respiratory difficulties (asphyxia, atelectasis, pneumonia and the respiratory distress syndrome; Comstock *et al.*, 1971; Andrews & McGarry, 1972; Meyer & Tonascia, 1977).

Complications of Pregnancy and Labour

Several complications of pregnancy and labour are associated with maternal smoking habits (Table 10.6). These trends persist after controlling for other risk factors such as parity and socio-economic status. Specifically identified hazards encountered by the smoking mother include bleeding during pregnancy, premature rupture of the membranes, placenta praevia and abruptio placentae (Underwood *et al.*, 1965; Russell *et al.*, 1966; Kullander & Kaellen, 1971; Andrews & McGarry, 1972; Cope *et al.*, 1973; Goujard *et al.*, 1975; Meyer & Tonascia, 1977; Naeye *et al.*, 1977). Such conditions make a substantial contribution to both the risk of premature delivery and the increased perinatal mortality found among the offspring of smoking mothers. In some instances (such as placenta praevia), the risk persists even if a woman stops smoking before becoming pregnant (Naeye, 1979).

One complication of pregnancy that is less frequent among smokers is pre-eclampsia (Underwood *et al.*, 1967; Duffus & MacGillivray, 1968;

Table 10.6: The Influence of Maternal Smoking Habits Upon Perinatal
Mortality and Complications of Pregnancy

Variable	Incidence per 1,000 births and smoking habit of mother (packs/day)		
	0	Less than 1	1 or more
Perinatal mortality	23	28	33
Bleeding during pregnancy	117	142	180
Rupture of membranes more than 48 hours before delivery	16	23	36
Rupture of membranes only at admission	30	39	45
Placenta praevia	6.4	8.2	13.1
Abruptio placentae	16	21	29

Source: Based on data from Meyer & Tonascia, 1977.

Kullander & Kaellen, 1971; Cope *et al.*, 1973; Palmgren *et al.*, 1973;
Hollingsworth *et al.*, 1976). This effect is independent of social class,
maternal weight or maternal weight gain, and is probably attributable
to the hypotensive action of thiocyanate, formed during detoxification
of cigarette smoke (Andrews & McGarry, 1972; Palmgren *et al.*, 1973).
Other possible factors reducing the likelihood of pre-eclampsia include
the smaller size of the baby and a lesser increase of maternal blood
volume (Pirani & MacGillivray, 1978). If toxaemia of pregnancy does
develop, the risks of prenatal mortality are nevertheless greater for the
smoker (22%) than for the non-smoker (9%; Duffus & MacGillivray,
1968; Russell *et al.*, 1968; Andrews & McGarry, 1972).

The average duration of gestation is not influenced materially
by maternal smoking, there is a 36 to 47% increased risk of premature
birth if the mother smokes (Andrews & McGarry, 1972; Fabia, 1973).
Indeed, between 11 and 14% of all premature births are probably
attributable to maternal smoking. Such births amount to only a small
fraction of the total birth rate, but nevertheless account for much of
the perinatal mortality (Meyer, 1977).

The perinatal risks of premature rupture of the membranes, placenta
praevia and abruptio placentae, although seen among smoking mothers
as a class, are all further increased if delivery occurs before the 36th
week of gestation (Meyer & Tonascia, 1977).

Long-term Effects

Several recent studies have indicated that the health of infants over the first year of life is poorer if the mother is a smoker. However, since most of the women concerned smoke both during pregnancy and after the child is born, it is difficult to determine whether the cause of the infant's ill-health is smoke exposure pre- or post-partum.

A study from northern Finland (Rantakallio, 1978b) distinguished perinatal mortality (defined above) from neonatal mortality (deaths in the first 28 days after birth) and post neonatal mortality (from 28 days to five years after birth). Perinatal deaths were 2.4% for non-smokers, 2.6% for light smokers and 3.3% for women who smoked more than ten cigarettes per day. Neonatal mortality was 0.88% for non-smokers, and 1.26% for smokers, while post-neonatal mortality figures were 0.39% for non-smokers and 1.11% for smokers. The children of smokers made more visits to the doctor, required more admissions to hospital and had longer average periods of hospital residence than the children of non-smokers. The prime reason for their poor health experience was a high incidence of respiratory disease. Subjects were matched for age, place of residence and marital status, so that socio-economic factors are unlikely to have been responsible for the observed differences. One particularly convincing argument is that the children born to a sub-group of women who stopped smoking during the final trimester of pregnancy fared as well as those born to non-smokers.

Rantakallio *et al.* (1979) also commented on a higher incidence of squint among the pre-school children of smokers (2.25%) compared to non-smokers (1.15%). Squint seemed to be associated with low birth weight and with other diseases of the central nervous system.

The association between the sudden infant death syndrome and maternal smoking (Steele & Langworth, 1966; Bergman & Wiesner, 1976; Naeye *et al.*, 1976; Schrauzer *et al.*, 1978) has already been noted (see Chapter 7). The experience of Bergman & Wiesner (1976) is fairly typical; they observed 61% of affected mothers smoked during pregnancy and 59% during the puerperium, compared with 42 and 42% in control subjects. Again, further investigation is needed to clarify whether the problem arises from smoking during or subsequent to pregnancy.

Table 10.7: Reported Percentage Reduction of Smoking During
Pregnancy

Per cent reduction %	Given smoking education %	Not given smoking education %
10–49	19	4
50	32	35
51–99	20	27
100	29	34

Source: Based on data from Langford *et al.*, 1980.

Table 10.8: Total Information on Smoking and Pregnancy in Toronto
Morning Paper[a] over Three-year Period

Date	Name of article	Area (cm²)
13 January 1978	'Study finds nicotine gathers in the breasts of women smokers'	250
17 January 1979	'Pre-pregnancy smoking harmful to fetus, US Researchers say'	84
12 June 1979	'Controversy being lit on health effect of breathing in second-hand smoke'[b]	440
19 September 1980	'Preconception health factors can affect fetus'[b]	390

Notes: a. Over the same period, the larger evening paper carried seven articles
mentioning smoking during pregnancy (some 5,700 cm² of information), while
the total coverage in 3 Canadian magazines was less than 2,000 cm² (one article
per magazine).
    b. Smoking, pregnancy and infant death were not the main foci of these
articles.
Source: Data collected in 1981 by Shephard & Lorimer, unpublished.

Attitudes of Women to Smoking During Pregnancy

Pregnancy is a critical life-event that provides a unique opportunity
for breaking the smoking habit. The attention of the mother becomes
focused upon the health of the developing fetus, and there are unique
opportunities for advice from health professionals as a series of antenatal
clinics are attended. Nevertheless, only a minority of women stop
smoking or even reduce their cigarette consumption during pregnancy
(Landesman-Dwyer & Emmanuel, 1979; Langford *et al.*, 1980; US
Surgeon General, 1980; Table 10.7). Occasional reports of greater
success (Donovan *et al.*, 1975; Baric *et al.*, 1976; Danaher *et al.*, 1978;
Gastrin & Ramstrom, 1979) must take account of volunteer status.

Table 10.9: Knowledge of Pregnant Women Concerning Effects of Smoking

Belief	Per cent agreeing
Baby will have smaller birthweight	35
Nicotine transmitted to breast milk	41
Parental smoking can affect baby's health	64
Parental example influences children's smoking	61

Source: Based on data from Langford *et al.*, 1980.

Table 10.10: Knowledge of Women Concerning the Effects of Smoking on Pregnancy

Belief	Never pregnant	Previously pregnant	Now pregnant	Smoked or will smoke in pregnancy
Smoking causes problems to unborn babies	83.3	93.8	100.0	100.0
Smoking causes problems to newborn babies	50.0	56.3	66.7	50.0
Smoking causes problems in child development	50.0	43.8	66.7	33.3

Source: Data collected in 1981 by Shephard & Lorimer, unpublished.

Table 10.11: Smoking Habits of Women Smokers One Year After Delivery

Situation	Per cent smoking
While caring for baby (feeding, bathing)	31
In baby's room	9
In mother's room	43
In the rest of the house	97
In the car with baby	65

Source: Based on data from Langford *et al.*, 1980.

Moreover, smoking withdrawal statistics must be viewed with scepticism unless objective measures of cigarette usage are obtained. Finally, a reduction in the number of cigarettes consumed per day, or in the number of 'puffs' taken per cigarette, does not necessarily lead to a reduced intake of nicotine and other harmful smoke constituents (Ashton, 1976; Gritz & Jarvik, 1978).

Since the half-time for the elimination of carbon monoxide from mother and fetus is only a few hours, there is merit in enforcing a ban on smoking for the critical period of delivery even if the mother has smoked throughout pregnancy (Davies *et al.*, 1981).

Despite very limited newspaper and magazine coverage of the topic (Table 10.8), a majority of young female smokers appreciate that their habit has a harmful effect upon the fetus and the newborn child (Yankelovich *et al.*, 1977; Langford *et al.*, 1980; Tables 10.9 and 10.10). Indeed, this is the commonest reason cited for a cessation of smoking during pregnancy. Fear of excessive weight gain is sometimes advanced as an argument against smoking withdrawal (Donovan *et al.*, 1975). Success of quitting depends on the firmness of the belief that smoking will harm the fetus, along with other factors encountered in general-purpose smoking withdrawal clinics (Dohrenwend & Dohrenwend, 1974).

Danaher (1978) commented that lack of knowledge about the effects of smoking on the fetus was still found among some physicians specializing in obstetrics and gynaecology; for instance, 23.6% of such physicians denied any relationship between maternal smoking and neonatal death. As might be anticipated, this ignorance was particularly marked among physicians who were themselves smokers. There was also a substantial gap between the intent of physicians to offer advice and the reality of accomplishment. Thus, 45% of physicians claimed to tell 'all' or 'almost all' of their patients to stop smoking or to reduce cigarette consumption, and a further 13% claimed to offer such advice to 'many' or 'most' of their patients. However, only 24% of US women pregnant between 1970 and 1975 remembered receiving such advice (Harris, 1979).

A survey of 353 public health agencies and similar organizations conducting prenatal classes in Canada (McRae & Choi-Lao, 1978) found smoking education was given in 82.7% of classes. Arguments against such instruction included lack of time, lack of material, fear of upsetting the mothers and reluctance of teachers who were themselves smokers. Only 23% of antenatal class teachers provided specific guidance on how to stop smoking, and only 21% considered themselves well-prepared to undertake such activity.

Factors influencing the success of educational programmes (Table 10.11) include an early start (preferably before the patient becomes pregnant; Donovan *et al.*, 1975), a high socio-economic status (Baric *et al.*, 1976), peer expectations (Baric & MacArthur, 1977), a history of previous birth complications (Danaher *et al.*, 1978) and person-to-person contact (Gastrin & Ramstrom, 1979).

11 FUTURE PROSPECTS

While it may be rash to speculate on the future course of passive exposure to cigarette smoke, it is nevertheless interesting to explore briefly a few likely developments.

Changes in Cigarette Design

Changes in cigarette design, aimed at reducing the health risk to the continuing smoker, are likely to continue (US Surgeon General, 1981). To the extent that improved combustion conditions reduce the output of tar and carbon monoxide, and variations of tobacco blend reduce the nicotine yield, these changes may be of incidental benefit to the non-smoker who is passively exposed to cigarette smoke.

On the other hand, cigarette manufacturers are now adding a wide range of secret flavouring agents to maintain the acceptability of their products to consumers, and the pyrolysis products of such additives may present a new hazard to the non-smoker. Moreover, while the tar and nicotine content of mainstream smoke is being reduced, there is no guarantee of similar changes in the composition of sidestream smoke (Aronow, 1978; Tager *et al.*, 1979; White & Froeb, 1980). Finally, a reduction in the nicotine yield per cigarette will probably encourage persistent smokers to consume a larger number of cigarettes per day, increasing the pollution of indoor air with other smoke constituents (Russell, 1980; Hill & Marquardt, 1980).

Cigarette Consumption

Current trends whereby the proportion of regular cigarette smokers is decreasing, but the consumption of individual smokers is increasing (British Medical Journal, 1981) seem likely to continue in Western Europe and North America. Nevertheless, the Scandinavian hope of educating a 'smoke-free generation' seems unlikely to be realised. Experience with other drugs of addiction such as cocaine and morphine has shown that despite wide public knowledge of the risks to health, a proportion of society will experiment to the point that they become habitual users.

157

Cigarette manufacturers in general seem reconciled to a long-term decrease of sales in Western Europe and North America, and have calculated very shrewdly that this challenge to their profits can be more than offset by implanting the cigarette habit in an increased proportion of the teeming millions living in the 'Third World'.

Taking a global perspective, the problem of passive smoking may thus show an increase rather than a decrease over the next 20 years. Moreover, in many Third World countries, crowded living conditions and apalling urban pollution will exacerbate the health hazards of passive smoke exposure relative to effects now perceived in Western society.

Problems of Air Pollution

Even in North America, the energy crisis is now threatening default on hard-won commitments to a cleaner environment. Reactivation of thermal generators fired by soft coal will greatly augment the atmospheric burden of particulate matter and oxides of sulphur, while rapidly escalating prices of petroleum will force a re-examination of techniques for restricting the carbon monoxide emission of automobiles. A general deterioration of urban air quality will certainly add to the risks of passive cigarette smoke exposure, and in some instances there may be a synergistic effect.

The energy crisis will also encourage the development of more airtight buildings, with reduced standards of ventilation, and this will require stringent control of all indoor pollutants, including cigarette smoke.

Problems of the Fetus

To date, the impact of maternal smoking has fallen most heavily upon very young mothers; however, this has probably been due mainly to related factors of social class. In the future, increased sophistication of contraception, world pressures of population and the economic necessity of a dual family income seem likely to cause a progressive rise of maternal age at delivery. To the extent that the oxygen supply of the fetus is more precarious in an older woman, the impact of smoking during pregnancy is thus likely to increase. This trend may be exacerbated by cigarettes with a low nicotine yield, since female addicts will be provoked to a higher daily cigarette consumption, and thus a higher carbon monoxide intake.

Future Research

There is little dispute that presently encountered ambient levels of cigarette smoke cause annoyance, irritation and visual symptoms in the majority of normal non-smokers. A proportion of non-smokers also experience nasal discharge or stuffiness, cough and sputum in badly contaminated areas. Exposure to cigarette smoke is thus harmful to 'health' as defined by the World Health Organisation, that is to say a condition characterized by the presence of full psychological, mental and social well-being (WHO, 1960). Whether such a definition of health can be legally enforced in disputes between smokers and non-smokers is more debatable.

Available information suggests that normal subjects develop minimal respiratory reactions when acutely exposed to accumulations of cigarette smoke. However, more research is needed on the response to aged cigarette smoke, and tests should also be conducted under conditions of vigorous exercise, where subjects are obliged to breathe the contaminated air via the mouth rather than the nose.

A proportion of subjects with asthma develop a wheezing reaction when they are exposed to cigarette smoke. Further study of this phenomenon is needed, but it appears to be a non-specific irritation of a sensitive airway rather than a true allergic reaction.

The main health concern arises from prolonged exposure to cigarette smoke. Further well-designed epidemiological surveys are required, but current evidence points to: (i) an increased incidence of respiratory disease in very young children; (ii) an increased risk of small airway disease in adults; and (iii) an increased risk of lung cancer. The litany of potential health effects is such that additional research is urgently needed. If the various allegations are upheld, the passive smoker is likely to become a militant non-smoker, prepared to take much stronger action to gain protection against involuntary exposure to cigarette smoke. It is arguable that a smoker has the right to destroy his own health, so long as the resultant medical costs are not charged to the community. However, there are no grounds for allowing the smoker to endanger the health of family, friends and colleagues.

REFERENCES

Abel, E.L. (1980) 'The fetal alcohol syndrome: behavioural teratology', *Psychol. Bull.*, *87*, 29–50

Adams, J.D., Erickson, H.H. & Stone, H.I. (1973) 'Myocardial metabolism during exposure to carbon monoxide in the conscious dog', *J. Appl. Physiol.*, *34*, 238–42

Alberman, E., Creasy, M., Elliott, M. & Spicer, C. (1976) 'Maternal factors associated with fetal chromosomal anomalies in spontaneous abortions', *Brit. J. Obstet. Gynecol.*, *83*, 621–7

American Conference of Government Industrial Hygienists. (1974) 'TLVs[®] threshold limit values for chemical substances in workroom air adopted by the American Conference of Government Industrial Hygienists for 1973', *J. Occup. Med.*, *16*, 39–49

Anderson, E.W., Andelman, R.J., Strauch, J.M., Fortuin, N.J. & Knelson, J.H. (1973) 'Effect of low-level carbon monoxide exposure on onset and duration of angina pectoris. A study in ten patients with ischemic heart disease', *Ann. Int. Med.*, *79*, 46–50

Anderson, E.W., Strauch, J., Knelson, J. & Fortuin, N. (1971) 'Effects of carbon monoxide (CO) on exercise electrocardiogram (ECG) and systolic time intervals (STI)', *Circulation*, *44*, Suppl. II, 135

Anderson, G. & Dalhamn, T. (1973) 'Hälsoriskerna vid passiv rökning', *Läkartidn*, *70*, 2833–6

Andrew, A.W. & Harriss, R.C. (1971) 'Mercury content of tobaccos', *Environ. Letters*, *1*, 231–4

Andrews, J. (1973) 'Thiocyanate and smoking in pregnancy', *Brit. J. Obstetr. Gynecol.*, *80*, 810–14

Andrews, J. & McGarry, J.M. (1972) 'A community study of smoking in pregnancy', *J. Obstetr. Gynecol. Brit. Commonw.*, *79*, 1057–73

Arfmann, B.L. & Chapanis, N.P. (1962) 'The relative sensitivities of taste and smell in smokers and non-smokers', *J. Gen. Psychol.*, *66*, 315–20

Armitage, A.K. (1965) 'Effects of nicotine and tobacco smoke on blood pressure and release of catecholamines from the adrenal glands', *Brit. J. Pharmac.*, *25*, 515–26

Armitage, A.K., Davies, R.F. & Turner, D.M. (1976) 'The effects of carbon monoxide on the development of atherosclerosis in the white carneau pigeon', *Atherosclerosis*, *23*, 333–44

Armitage, A.K., Dollery, C.T., George, C.F., Houseman, T.H., Lewis, P.J. & Turner, D.M. (1975) 'Absorption and metabolism of nicotine from cigarettes', *Brit. Med. J.*, *4*, 313–16

Armitage, A.K., Dollery, C.T., Houseman, T., Kohner, E., Lewis, P.J. & Turner, D. (1978) 'Absorption of nicotine from small cigars', *Clin. Pharm. Therap.*, *23*, 143–51

Armitage, A.K. & Turner, D.M. (1970) 'Absorption of nicotine in cigarette and cigar smoke through the oral mucosa', *Nature*, *226*, 1231–2

Armstrong, H.E. (1922) 'Carbonic oxide in tobacco smoke', *Brit. Med. J.*, (*i*), 992–3

Aronow, W.S. (1974) 'Effects of passive smoking on angina pectoris', *New Engl. J. Med.*, *299*, 21–4

———— (1978) 'Effects of passive smoking on angina pectoris', *New Engl. J. Med.*, *299*, 21–4

Aronow, W.S., Cassidy, J., Vangrow, J.S., March, H., Kern, J.C., Goldsmith, J.R., Khemka, M., Pagano, J. & Vawter, M. (1974) 'Effect of cigarette smoking and breathing carbon monoxide on cardiovascular hemodynamics in anginal patients', *Circulation, 50*, 340-7

Aronow, W.S., Ferlinz, J. & Glauser, F. (1977) 'Effect of carbon monoxide on exercise performance in chronic obstructive pulmonary disease', *Amer. J. Med., 63*, 904-8

Aronow, W.S., Harris, C.N., Isbell, M.W., Rokaw, S.N. & Imparato, B. (1972) 'Effect of freeway travel on angina pectoris', *Ann. Intern. Med., 77*, 669-76

Aronow, W.S. & Isbell, M.W. (1973) 'Carbon monoxide: effect on exercise-induced angina pectoris', *Ann. Intern. Med., 79*, 392-5

Ashe, W.F. (1952) 'Acute effects of air pollution in Donora, Pa.', *Proc. U.S. Tech. Conf. on Air Pollution*, McGraw Hill, New York, pp. 455-61

Ashton, H. (1976) 'Effect of smoking on carboxyhaemoglobin level in pregnancy', *Brit. Med. J., 1*, 42-3

Asmussen, I. (1977) 'Ultrastructure of the human placenta at term. Observations on placentas from newborn children of smoking and non-smoking mothers', *Acta Obstetr. Gynecol. Scand., 56*, 119-26

———— (1978) 'Ultrastructure of human umbilical veins', *Acta Obstet. Gynecol. Scand., Suppl. 57*, 253-5

Asmussen, I. & Kjeldsen, K. (1975) 'Intimal ultrastructure of human umbilical arteries. Observations on arteries from newborn children of smoking and non-smoking mothers', *Circ. Res., 36*, 579-89

Åstrup, P. (1969) 'Effects of hypoxia and of carbon monoxide exposures on experimental atherosclerosis', *Ann. Int. Med., 71*, 426-7

Åstrup, P., Olsen, H.K., Trolle, D. & Kjeldsen, K. (1972) 'Effect of moderate carbon monoxide exposure on fetal development', *Lancet, 2*, 1220-2

Aviado, D.M., Samanek, M. & Folle, L.E. (1966) 'Cardiopulmonary effects of tobacco and related substances. 1. The release of histamine during inhalation of cigarette smoke and anoxaemia in the heart-lung and intact dog preparation', *Arch. Env. Health, 12*, 705-11

Ayres, C.I. & Thornton, R.E. (1965) 'Determination of benzo (α) pyrene and related compounds in cigarette smoke', *Beitr. Tabakforsch., 3*, 285-90

Ayres, S.M., Giannelli, S. & Armstrong, R.G. (1965) 'Carboxyhemoglobin: hemodynamic and respiratory responses to small concentrations', *Science, 149*, 193-4

Ayres, S.M., Giannelli, S. & Mueller, H. (1970) 'Myocardial and systemic responses to carboxyhemoglobin', *Ann. N.Y. Acad. Sci., 174*, 268-93

Ayres, S.M., Mueller, H.S., Gregory, J.J., Giannelli, S. & Penny, J.L. (1969) 'Systemic and myocardial hemodynamic responses to relatively small concentrations of carboxyhemoglobin (COHb)', *Arch. Environ. Health, 18*, 699-709

Ayres, S.M., Penny, J., Criscitiello, A. & Giannelli, S. (1968) 'Effect of abnormal hemoglobin (carboxyhemoglobin) on human myocardial metabolism', *Clin. Res., 16*, 220

Bahna, S.L. & Bjerkedal, T. (1975) 'Smoking and intraocular pressure', *Acta Ophthalmol., 53*, 328-34

Bailey, R.R. (1970) 'The effect of maternal smoking on the infant birth weight', *N.Z. Med. J., 71*, 293-4

Baird, D. (1964) 'The epidemiology of prematurity', *J. Pediatr., 65*, 909-24

Baker, M. & McKendrick, S. (1976) 'Legislation and smoking. Project 1216-5-100', *Ontario Interagency Council on Smoking*, September 1976

Baker, R.R. (1974) 'Temperature distribution inside a burning cigarette', *Nature, 247*, 405-6

Ballantyne, J.W. (1902) *Manual of antenatal pathology and hygiene. The fetus*, William Green & Sons, Edinburgh.

Baric, L. & MacArthur, C. (1977) 'Health norms in pregnancy', *Brit. J. Prev. Soc. Med.*, *31*, 30–8

Baric, L., MacArthur, C. & Sherwood, M. (1976) 'A study of health education aspects of smoking in pregnancy', *Int. J. Health Ed.*, *Suppl. 19*, 1–16

Bartlett, O. (1968) 'Patho-physiology of exposure to low concentrations of CO', *Arch. Environ. Health*, *16*, 719–27

Basu, P.K., Lusis, G. & Dhurandhar, R. (1971) 'The effect of air pollutants on the eye. II. A study of their effect on the oculocardiac reflex', *Canad. J. Ophthalmol.*, *6*, 136–8

Basu, P.K., Pimm, P.E., Shephard, R.J. & Silverman, F. (1978) 'The effect of cigarette smoke on the human tear film', *Canad. J. Ophthalmol.*, *13*, 22–6

Baumberger, J.P. (1923) 'The amount of smoke produced from tobacco and its absorption in smoking as determined by electrical precipitation', *J. Pharmacol. Ther.*, *21*, 47–57

Beard, R.R. & Grandstaff, N.W. (1970) 'Carbon monoxide exposure and cerebral function', *Ann. N.Y. Acad. Sci.*, *174*, 385–95

———— (1972) 'Carbon monoxide and human functions', paper presented at 5th Rochester International Conference on Environmental Toxicity: Behavioral Toxicology, 7–9 June 1972

Beard, R.R. & Wertheim, G.A. (1967) 'Behavioral impairment associated with small doses of carbon monoxide', *Amer. J. Publ. Health*, *57*, 2012–22

Beaver, H. (1954) 'Mortality and morbidity during the London fog of December 1952', *Reports on Public Health and Medical Subjects*, *95*, 1–61

Becker, C.G. & Dubin, T. (1977) 'Activation of Factor XII by tobacco glycoprotein', *J. Exp. Med.*, *146*, 457–67

Behr, M.J., Leong, K.H. & Jones, R.H. (1981) 'Acute effects of cigarette smoking on left ventricular function at rest and exercise', *Med. Sci. Sports Exercise*, *13*, 9–12

Bender, W., Gothert, M., Malorny, G. & Sebbesse, P. (1971) 'Wirkungsbild niedriger Kohlenoxid-Konzentratisnen beim Menschen', *Archiv. für Toxikol.*, *27*, 142–58

Bentley, H.R. & Burgan, J.G. (1961) Cited by E.L. Wynder & Hoffmann (1967). *Tobacco Manufacturers' Standing Committee Research Papers 4*, 2nd edn

Bergman, A.B. & Wiesner, L.A. (1976) 'Relationship of passive cigarette smoking to sudden infant death syndrome', *Pediatrics*, *58*, 665–8

Bernhard, P. (1962) 'Die Wirkung des Rauchens auf Frau und Mutter', *Soz. Ned. Hyg.*, *104*, 1826–31

Bhargava, S.K. (1973) 'Tobacco amblyopia and acquired dyschromatopsia anomaloscope tests', *Acta Ophthalmol.*, *51*, 822–8

Birstingl, M., Hawkins, L. & McEwen, T. (1970) 'Experimental atherosclerosis during chronic exposure to carbon monoxide', *Europ. Surg. Res.*, *2*, 92–3

Bisdom, C.J.W. (1937) 'Alcohol en nicotinever giftigung bij zuigelingen', *Maandschr. v. Kindergeneeskunde*, *6*, 332–41

Blackburn, H., Brozek, J. & Taylor, H.L. (1960) 'Common circulatory measurements in smokers and non-smokers', *Circulation*, *22*, 1112–24

Blake, C.A. & Sawyer, C.H. (1972) 'Nicotine blocks the suckling-induced rise in circulating prolactin in lactating rats', *Science*, *177*, 619–21

Blue, J.A. (1970) 'Cigarette asthma and allergy', *Ann. Allergy*, *28*, 110–15

Bocca, E. & Battiston, M.N. (1964) 'Odour perception and environment conditions', *Acta Otolaryngol.*, *57*, 391–400

Boex, A. (1972) 'Gesetzesgebung und Rauchen', *Rehabilitation Praventivmedizin Physikalische Medizin, Sozialmedizin*, *25*, 46–8

Bogen, E. (1929) 'The composition of cigarets and cigaret smoke', *J. Amer. Med. Assoc.*, *93*, 1110-14

Bonham, G.H. (1973) 'Fasten your seat belts – no smoking', *Brit. Col. Med. J.*, *15*, 304-5

Borlee, I. & Lechat, M.F. (1979) 'Resultats d'une enquête sur les malformations congenitales dans le Hainaut', *Belg. Med. Soc. Hyg.*, *36*, 77-99

Boren, H.G. (1970) 'Pulmonary cell kinetics after exposure to cigarette smoke' in M.G. Hanna, P. Nettesheim & J.R. Gilbert (eds.), *Inhalation Carcinogenesis*, US Atomic Energy Commission, Oakridge, Tenn., pp. 229-41

Bouhuys, A. (1977) 'Lung diseases in rural and urban communities', *National Heart, Lung & Blood Institute*, Bethesda, Md., PB-267-974, pp. 1-98

Bradt, P.T. & Herrenkohl, R.C. (1976) 'DDT in human milk. What determines the levels?', *Sci. Total Environ.*, *6*, 161-3

Brandt, E. & Matczynski, M.J. (1976) 'This is clean indoor air country', *Amer. Lung Assoc. Bull.*, *62*, 11-13

Bridge, D.P. & Corn, M. (1972) 'Contribution to the assessment of exposure of non-smokers to air pollution from cigarette and cigar smoke in occupied spaces', *Environ. Res.*, *5*, 192-209

Bridges, B.A., Chelmmesen, J. & Sugimura, T. (1979) 'Cigarette smoking – does it carry a genetic risk?', *Mutation Res.*, *65*, 71-81

British Medical Journal (1978a) 'Cigarette smoking and spontaneous abortion' (editorial), *Brit. Med. J.*, (*i*), 259-60

——— (1978b) 'Breathing other people's smoke' (editorial), *Brit. Med. J.*, (*ii*), 453-4

——— (1981) 'Ten years of ASH' (editorial), *Brit. Med. J.*, *282*, 340-1

Broder, I., Higgins, M.W., Mathews, K.P. & Keller, J.B. (1974) 'Epidemiology of asthma and allergic rhinitis in a total community, Tecumseh, Michigan. III. Second survey of the community', *J. Allergy Clin. Immunol.*, *53*, 127-38

Brody, J.A. (1977) 'To permit or prohibit smoking in high schools: its a burning issue', *Amer. School Board J.*, *164*, 19-21

Brown, A. (1923) 'Present day treatment of asthma', *New York Med. J. & Med. Rev.*, *98*, 333-6

Brunnemann, K.D. & Hoffmann, D. (1974) 'Chemical studies on tobacco smoke XXIV. A quantitative method for carbon monoxide and carbon dioxide in cigarette and cigar smoke', *J. Chromat. Sci.*, *12*, 70-5

Brunnemann, K.D., Yu, L. & Hoffmann, D. (1977a) In: World Smoking and Health 2, 23

——— (1977b) 'Assessment of carcinogenic volatile N-nitrosamines in tobacco and in mainstream and sidestream smoke from cigarettes', *Cancer Res.*, *37*, 3218-22

——— (1977c) 'Chemical studies on tobacco XLIX. Gas chromatographic determination of hydrogen cyanide and cyanogen in tobacco smoke', *J. Analyt. Toxicol.*, *1*, 38-42

Bulay, O.M. & Wattenberg, L.W. (1970) 'Carcinogenic effects of sub-cutaneous administration of benzo (α) pyrene during pregnancy on the progeny', *Proc. Soc. Exp. Biol. Med.*, *135*, 84-6

Buncher, C.R. (1969) 'Cigarette smoking and duration of pregnancy', *Amer. J. Obst. Gynecol.*, *103*, 942-6

Buratowski, J., Warczynski, A. & Piasecki, M. (1974) 'Wplyw Malych Stezen Nikotyna Zdolnosc Adaptacjii i Ostrosc Wzroku u Ludzi nie Palacych Tytoniu'. (The effect of small concentrations of nicotine on the ability of visual adaptation and acuity in non-smokers), *Polski Tygodnik Lekarski*, *29* (25), 1077-8

Burn, J.H. (1960) 'The action of nicotine on the peripheral circulation', *Ann.*

N.Y. Acad. Sci., *90*, 81–4

Burns, D.M. (1977) 'Consequences of smoking – the involuntary smoker' in *Health Consequences, Education, Cessation Activities and Governmental Action. Vol. II. Proceedings of the 3rd World Conference on Smoking and Health. New York June 2–5, 1975*, National Institutes of Health, Bethesda, Md., DHEW Publication 77–1413

Busey, W.M. (1972) *Summary report: study of synergistic effects of certain airborne systems in the cynomagus monkey*, Hazelton Laboratories, Inc., Vienna, Va.

Butler, N.R. & Alberman, E.D. (1969) *Perinatal problems. The second report of the 1958 British perinatal mortality survey*, E.S. Livingstone, Edinburgh

Butler, N.R. & Goldstein, H. (1973) 'Smoking in pregnancy and subsequent child development', *Brit. Med. J.*, *4*, 573

Calvet, J. & Coll, J. (1968) 'Le cancer dans les maladies professionnelles en oto-rhino-laryngologie', *Arch. Mal. Prof.*, *29*, 516–19

Cameron, P. (1972) 'Second-hand tobacco smoke: children's reactions', *J. School Health*, *42*, 280–4

Cameron, P., Kostin, J.S., Zaks, J.M., Wolfe, J.H., Tighe, G., Oselett, B., Stocker, R. & Winton, J. (1969) 'The health of smokers' and non-smokers' children', *J. Allergy*, *43*, 336–41

Cameron, P. & Robertson, D. (1973) 'Effect of home environment tobacco smoke on family health', *J. Appl. Psychol.*, *57*, 142–7

Camner, P., Philipson, K. & Arvidsson, T. (1971) 'Cigarette smoking in man', Short-term *Arch. Env. Health*, *23*, 421–6

——— (1973) 'Withdrawal of cigarette smoking: a study on tracheobronchial clearance', *A.M.A. Arch. Env. Health*, *26*, 90–2

Campbell, D. (1976) 'Smoking policies in hospitals', *Dimensions in Health Service*, *53*, 20–3

Campbell, J.M. & Lindsey, A.J. (1957) 'Polycyclic hydrocarbons in cigar smoke', *Brit. J. Cancer*, *11*, 192–5

Cano, J.P., Catalin, J., Badre, R., Dumas, C., Viala, A. & Guillerme, R. (1970) 'Determination de la nicotine par chromatographie en phase gazeuse II', *Ann. Pharm. Franç.*, *28*, 633–40

Carpenter, R.D., Gager, F.L. & Jenkins, R.W. (1970) Paper presented at 24th Tobacco Chemists Research Conference, Montreal, P.Q., Oct. 28–30th, 1970

Carter, W.L. & Hasegawa, I. (1975) 'Fixation of tobacco smoke aerosols for size distribution studies', *J. Colloid Interface Sci.*, *53*, 134–41

Center for Disease Control (1978) *State legislation on smoking and health, 1978*, US Dept. of Health, Education and Welfare, Public Health Service, Center for Disease Control, DHEW Publication CDC 79–8331

Chappell, S.B. & Parker, R.J. (1977) 'Smoking and carbon monoxide levels in enclosed public places in New Brunswick', *Canad. J. Publ. Health*, *68*, 159–61

Chase, H.C. (1969) 'Infant mortality and weight at birth: 1960 United States birth cohort', *Amer. J. Publ. Hlth*, *59*, 1618–28

Cherniack, R.M. (1977) 'Smoking and chronic airways obstruction', *National Heart, Lung and Blood Institute, Division of Lung Diseases*, Bethesda, Md., Nat. Tech. Inf. Service PB 272–154, pp. 1–41

Chevalier, R.B., Bowers, J.A., Bondurant, S. & Ross, J.C. (1963) 'Circulatory and ventilatory effects of exercise in smokers and non-smokers', *J. Appl. Physiol.*, *18*, 357–60

Chisholm, I.A. (1971) 'The dyschromatopsia of pernicious anaemia', *Mod. Probl. Ophthalmol.*, *11*, 130–5

Chisholm, I.A., Bronte-Stewart, J. & Awduche, E.O. (1971) 'Colour vision in tobacco amblyopia', *Acta Ophthalmol.*, *48*, 1145–56

Chobot, R. (1934) 'The significance of tobacco reactions in allergic children', *J. Allergy*, *6*, 383–6

Christianson, R.E. (1979) 'Gross differences observed in the placentas of smokers and non-smokers', *Amer. J. Epidemiol.*, *110*, 178–87

Chu, Y.M., Parlett, R.C. & Wright, G.L. (1970) 'A preliminary investigation of some immunological aspects of tobacco use', *Amer. Rev. Resp. Dis.*, *102*, 118–23

Chyle, P., Chyle, M. & Patocka, F. (1971) 'Virus tabakove mozaiky a polyfenoly jako priorozene se vyskytujici kancerogeny v Tabaku', *Casopis Lekaru Ceskych*, *110*, 189–90

Civil Aeronautics Board (US) (1973) *Part 252 – Provision of designated "No-Smoking" areas aboard aircraft operated by certificated air carriers*, US Civil Aeronautics Board, Regulation ER 800, pp. 1–8

Clark, B.J. & Coburn, R.F. (1975) 'Mean myoglobin tension during exercise at maximal oxygen uptake', *J. Appl. Physiol.*, *39*, 135–44

Clarke, B.G., Guyatt, A.R. & Alpers, J.H. (1970) 'Changes in airway conductance on smoking a cigarette', *Thorax*, *25*, 418–22

Coburn, R.F. (1977) 'The biological effects of carbon monoxide on the human organism', *Report of a Committee on the National Research Council – National Academy of Sciences*, US National Academy of Sciences and Environmental Protection Agency, Washington, DC

Cockcroft, D.W., MacCormack, D.W., Tarlo, S.M., Hargreave, F.E. & Pengelly, L.D. (1979) 'Nasal airway inspiratory resistance', *Amer. Rev. Resp. Dis.*, *119*, 921–6

Cohen, S.I., Deane, M. & Goldsmith, J.R. (1969) 'Carbon monoxide and survival from myocardial infarction', *Arch. Env. Health*, *19*, 510–17

Colley, J.R.T. (1974) 'Respiratory symptoms in children and parental smoking and phlegm production', *Brit. Med. J.*, *2*, 201–4

Colley, J.R.T., Holland, W.W. & Corkhill, R.T. (1974) 'Influence of passive smoking and parental phlegm on pneumonia and bronchitis in early childhood', *Lancet*, *2* (7888), 1031–4

Commins, B.T. (1975) 'Measurement of carbon monoxide in the blood: review of available methods', *Ann. Occup. Hyg.*, *18*, 69–77

Commins, B.T. & Lawther, P.J. (1965) 'A sensitive method for the determination of carboxyhaemoglobin in a finger prick sample of blood', *Brit. J. Industr. Med.*, *22*, 139–43

Comroe, J.S. (1964) 'The physiological effects of smoking', *Physiology for Physicians*, *2*, 1–6

Comstock, G.W. & Lundin, F.E. (1967) 'Parental smoking and perinatal mortality', *Amer. J. Obst. Gynecol.*, *98*, 708–18

Comstock, G.W., Shah, F.K., Meyer, M.B. & Abbey, H. (1971) 'Low birth weight and neonatal mortality rate related to maternal smoking on socioeconomic status', *Amer. J. Obstet. Gynecol.*, *111*, 53–9

Conraux, C. & Collard, M. (1975) 'La modification du nystagmus sous l'effet des drogues médicamenteuses', *Acta Oto-Rhino-Laryngologica Belg.*, *29*, 113–22

Cope, I., Lancaster, P. & Stevens, L. (1973) 'Smoking in pregnancy', *Med. J. Austral.*, *1*, 73–7

Corbaz, R., Artho, A., Ceschini, P., Häusermann, M. & Plantefève, J.C.I. (1969) 'Herbicide residues in tobacco leaves and their transfer into the smoke. Urea herbicides, Patoran and Molipan', *Beitr. Tabakforsch.*, *5*, 80–91

Covert, D.S. & Frank, N.R. (1980) 'Atmospheric particles. Behavior and functional effects', in J.A. Nadel (ed.), *Physiology and pharmacology of the airways*, Dekker, New York, pp. 259–95

Crews, S.J., James, B., Marsters, J.B. & West, R.H. (1970) 'Drug and nutritional factors in optic neuropathy', *Trans. Ophthalm. Soc. U.K.*, *90*, 773–94

Crofton, E.C., Hawthorne, V.M. & Hedley, A.J. (1977) 'Smoking in Scottish hospitals. An ASH survey', *Health Bulletin*, *35*, 29–36

Croker, E.C. & Henderson, L.F. (1927) 'Analysis and classification of odors', *Amer. Perfum. Essent. Oil Rev.*, *22*, 325–7

Cropp, G.J.A. (1970) 'Ventilation in anemia and polycythemia', *Can. J. Physiol. Pharm.*, *48*, 382–93

Crosby, W.M., Metcoff, J., Costiloe, J.P., Mameesh, M., Sandstead, H.H., Jacob, R.A., McClain, P.E., Jacobson, G., Reid, W. & Burns, G. (1977) 'Fetal malnutrition: an appraisal of correlated factors', *Amer. J. Obstetr. Gynecol.*, *128*, 22–31

Cryer, P.E., Haymond, M.W., Santiago, J.V. & Shah, S.D. (1976) 'Norepinephrine and epinephrine release and adrenergic mediation of smoking-associated haemodynamic and metabolic events', *New Engl. J. Med.*, *295*, 573–7

Cuddeback, J.E., Donovan, J.R. & Burg, W.R. (1976) 'Occupational aspects of passive smoking', *Amer. Industr. Hyg. Assoc. J.*, *37*, 263–7

Curphey, T.J., Hood, L.P.L. & Perkins, N.M. (1965) 'Carboxyhemoglobin in relation to air pollution and smoking', *Arch. Environ. Health*, *10*, 179–85

Daff, M.E. & Kennaway, E.L. (1950) 'The arsenic content of tobacco and of tobacco smoke', *Brit. J. Cancer*, *4*, 173–82

Dahlström, H. (1955) 'A critical study of Sjöstrand's method for determination of COHb and the total hemoglobin of the human body', *Acta Physiol. Scand.*, *33*, 296–308

Dalhamn, T. (1966) 'Effect of cigarette smoke on ciliary activity', *Amer. Rev. Resp. Dis.*, *93*, 108–14

Dalhamn, T., Edfors, M.L. & Rylander, R. (1968a) 'Mouth absorption of various compounds in cigarette smoke', *Arch. Environ. Health*, *16*, 831–5

―――― (1968b) 'Retention of cigarette smoke components in human lungs', *Arch. Env. Health*, *17*, 746–8

Danaher, B.G. (1978) 'Ob-Gyn intervention in helping smokers quit' in J.L. Schwartz (ed.), *Progress in Smoking Cessation*, Amer. Cancer Soc., New York, pp. 316–28

Danaher, B.G., Shisslak, C.M., Thompson, C.B. & Ford, J.D. (1978) 'A smoking cessation program for pregnant women: an explanatory study', *Amer. J. Publ. Health*, *68*, 896–8

DaSilva, A.M.T. & Hamosh, P. (1973) 'Effects of smoking a single cigarette on the "small airways"', *J. Appl. Physiol.*, *34*, 361–5

Dastur, D.K., Quadros, E.V., Wadia, N.H., Desai, M.M. & Bharvcha, E.D. (1972) 'Effect of vegetarianism and smoking on vitamin B_{12}, thiocyanate and folate levels in blood of normal subjects', *Brit. Med. J.*, *(ii)*, 260–3

Dautrebande, L. & Dubois, A.B. (1958) 'Acute effect of breathing inert dust particles and of carbachol aerosol on the mechanical characteristics of the lungs in man. Changes in response after inhaling sympathomimetic aerosols', *J. Clin. Invest.*, *37*, 1746–55

Davies, D.P., Gray, O.P., Ellwood, P.C. & Abernethy, M. (1976) 'Cigarette smoking in pregnancy: associations with maternal weight gain and fetal growth', *Lancet*, *(i)*, 385–7

Davies, J.H., Latto, I.P., Jones, J.G., Veale, A. & Wardrop, C.A.J. (1981) 'The effects of stopping smoking for 48 hours on oxygen availability from the blood: a study in pregnant women', *Brit. Med. J.*, *2*, 355–6

Davis, K.M. (1975) 'Connecticutt works with health professionals', *Amer. Lung Assoc. Bull.*, *61*, 14 (May 1975)

DeBias, D.A., Banerjee, C.M., Birkhead, N.C., Grune, C.H., Scott, D. & Harrer, W.V. (1976) 'Effects of carbon monoxide inhalation on ventricular fibrillation', *Arch. Environ. Health, 31*, 38–42

Denson, P.M., Davidow, B., Bass, H.E. & Jones, E.W. (1967) 'A chemical test for smoking exposure', *Arch. Environ. Health, 14*, 865–74

Denson, R., Nanson, J.L. & McWatters, M.A. (1975) 'Hyperkinesis and maternal smoking', *Canad. Psychiatr. Assoc. J., 20*, 183–7

DeRouane, A. & Verduyn, G. (1974) 'Etude de quelques facteurs influencant la pollution de l'air à l'interieur des batiments', *Tribune de Cebedeau, 27*, 482–8

Dinman, B.D. (1968) 'Pathophysiologic determinants of community air quality standards for carbon monoxide', *J. Occup. Med., 10*, 446–56

Dohlman, C.H., Friend, J., Kalevar, B., Yagoda, D. & Balazs, E. (1976) 'The glycoprotein (mucus) content of tears from normal and dry eye patients', *Exp. Eye Res., 22*, 359–65

Dohrenwend, B.S. & Dohrenwend, D.P. (1974) *Stressful life events: their nature and effect*, John Wiley, New York

Donovan, J.R., Burgess, P.L., Hossack, C.M. & Yudkin, G.D. (1975) 'Routine advice against smoking in pregnancy', *J. Roy. Coll. Gen. Pract., 25*, 264–8

Dontenwill, W. & Wiebecke, B. (1966) 'Tracheal and pulmonary alterations following the inhalation of cigarette smoke by the golden hamster' in L. Severi (ed.), *Lung Tumours in Animals*, Univ. of Perugia, Division of Cancer Research, pp. 519–26

Dorman, R.G. (1971) 'Protection against dusts' in C.N. Davies (ed.), *Design and use of respirators*, Pergamon, New York, pp. 12–23

Dosman, J., Bode, F., Urbanette, J., Martin, R. & Macklem, P.T. (1975) 'The use of helium-oxygen mixture during maximum expiratory flow to demonstrate obstruction in small airways in smokers', *J. Clin. Invest., 55*, 1090–9

Dowdell, W. (1973/4) 'Non-smokers' revolt accelerates', *Cancer News, 27*, 2–4

Downing, G.C. & Chapman, W.E. (1966) 'Smoking and pregnancy. A statistical study of 5,659 patients', *Calif. Med., 104*, 187

Dravineks, A. & Krotoszynsky, B.K. (1966) 'Collection and processing of airborne chemical information', *J. Gas Chromatog., 4*, 367–70

Drinkwater, B.L., Raven, P.B., Horvath, S.M., Gliner, J.A., Ruhling, R.O., Bolduan, N.W. & Taguchi, S. (1974) 'Effect of carbon monoxide and peroxyacetyl nitrate on man's ability to work in the heat', *Arch. Environ. Health, 28*, 177–81

Dublin, W.B. (1972) 'Secondary smoking: a problem that deserves attention', *Pathologist, 26*, 244–5

Dudley, W.L. (1888) 'The poisonous effects of cigarette smoking', *Medical News, 53*, 286–8

Duffus, G.M. & MacGillivray, I. (1968) 'The incidence of pre-eclamptic toxemia in smokers and non-smokers', *Lancet, (1)*, 994–5

Dunn, H.G., McBurney, A.K., Ingram, S. & Hunter, C.M. (1976) 'Maternal cigarette smoking during pregnancy and the child's subsequent development: I. Physical growth to the age of 6½years', *Canad. J. Publ. Health, 67*, 499–505

—— (1977) 'Maternal cigarette smoking during pregnancy and the child's subsequent development: II. Neurological and intellectual maturation to the age of 6½ years', *Canad. J. Publ. Health, 68*, 43–50

Durazzini, G., Zazo, F. & Bertoni, G. (1975) 'The importance of the dosage of thiocyanates in urine and blood of flying personnel for the prevention of diseases of visual function' in G. Perdriel (ed.), *Medical requirements and examination procedures in relation to the tasks of today's aircrew: evaluation of the special senses for flying adults*, NATO Advisory Group for Aerospace Research and Development, Conference Proceedings 152 A7-1 to A7-5

Dwyer, W.F. (1978) 'Smoking: free choice', *Business Horizons, 21*, 52-6

Dyer, R.S., Eccles, C.U., Schwartzwelder, H.S., Fechter, L.D. & Annau, Z. (1979) 'Prenatal carbon monoxide and adult evoked potentials in rats', *J. Env. Sci. Hlth., C13*, 107-20

Eberle, A. (1977) 'Rechtliche Aspekte und Akzente des Passiv rauchens. Interdisciplinare Dekanstosse. Teil. 2. Die Aktivitat der Passiv-raucher – ihr Einstieg in die Forensische Praxis', *Therapie der Gegenwart, 116*, 1984-2000

Ebert, R.V. & Terracio, M.J. (1975) 'The bronchiolar epithelium in cigarette smokers', *Amer. Rev. Resp. Dis., 111*, 4-11

Egerton, A., Gugan, K. & Weinberg, F.J. (1936) *Combustion Flame, 7*, 63-78

Ekblom, B. & Huot, R. (1972) 'Response to submaximal and maximal exercise at different levels of carboxyhemoglobin', *Acta Physiol. Scand., 86*, 474-82

Elfinova, E.V., Gusev, M.I., Nokivov, J.V., Judina, T.V. & Sergiev, A.N. (1972) 'Study of the combined systemic effect of atmospheric pollutants (gases and dusts)', *Gig. Sanit., 8*, 11-15

Elmenhorst, H. & Schultz, C.H. (1968) 'Flüchtige Inhaltsstoffe des Tabakrauches, Die chemischen Bestandteile der Gas Dampf-Phase', *Beitr. Tabakforsch, 4*, 90-123

Emanuel, W. (1931) 'Über das Vorkommen von Nicotin in der Frauenmilch nach Zigarettengenub', *Z. Kinderh., 52*, 41-6

Emele, J.F. (1975) 'Pharmacology of nicotine' in J. Steinfeld, W. Griffiths, K. Ball & R.M. Taylor (eds.), *Proceedings of the Third World Conference on Smoking and Health, New York, June 2-5, Vol. II. Health consequences, education, cessation activities and social action*, US Dept. of Health, Education and Welfare, Public Health Service, Nat. Institutes of Health, National Cancer Institute, DHEW Publication 77-1413, pp. 561-7

Essenberg, J.M. (1952) 'Cigarette smoke and the incidence of primary neoplasm of the lung in the albino mouse', *Science, 116*, 561-2

Essenberg, J.M., Schwind, J.V. & Patras, A.B. (1940) 'The effects of nicotine and cigarette smoke on pregnant female albino rats and their offsprings', *J. Lab. Clin. Med., 25*, 708-17

Fabia, J. (1973) 'Cigarettes pendant la grossesse, poids de naissance et mortalité', *Canad. Med. Assoc. J., 109*, 1104-9

Falk, H.L. (1977) 'Chemical agents in cigarette smoke' in D.H.K. Lee (ed.), *Handbook of Physiology, Section 9 – Reactions to Environmental Agents*, Amer. Physiol. Soc., Washington, DC, pp. 199-211

Farago, L. (1968) 'Bericht uber Oto-Rhino-Laryngologische Krebsreihen-untersuchungen', *Monatsschrift für Ohrenheilkunde und Laryngo – Rhinologie, 102*, 588-601

Fechter, L.D. & Annau, Z. (1977) 'Toxicity of mild prenatal carbon monoxide exposure', *Science, 197*, 680-2

Federal Aviation Administration (1971) *Health aspects of smoking in transport aircraft*, US Dept. of Health, Education and Welfare, Public Health Service, Health Services and Mental Health Administration, Nat. Inst. Occup. Safety & Health, December 1971, pp. 1-85

Federal Register (1976) 'Smoking in GSA controlled building and facilities: guidelines', *Federal Register, 41* (197), 8 October 1976, 44424

——— (1979) 'Management of buildings and grounds: revision of building rules and regulations', *Federal Register, 44*, 16 April 1979, 22464-5

Fedrick, J. (1978) 'Factors associated with low birth weight of infants delivered in term', *Brit. J. Obstetr. Gynecol., 85*, 1-7

Ferguson, B.B., Wilson, D.J. & Schaffner, W. (1976) 'Determination of nicotine concentrations in human milk', *Amer. J. Dis. Childr., 130*, 837-9

Fergusson, D.M. (1979) 'Smoking during pregnancy', *New Z. Med. J., 89*, 41-3

Feron, V.J., Kruysse, A., Til, H.P. & Immel, H.R. (1978) 'Repeated exposure to acrolein vapour: subacute studies in hamsters, rats and rabbits', *Toxicology*, *9*, 47–57

Ferri, E.S. & Baratta, E.J. (1966) 'Polonium^{210} in tobacco, cigarette smoke, and selected human organs', *Public Health Rep.*, *81*, 121–7

Fielding, J.E. & Yankauer, A. (1978) 'The pregnant smoker', *Amer. J. Publ. Health*, *68*, 835–6

Fine, D.H., Rufeh, F., Lieb, D. & Rounbehler, D.P. (1975) 'Description of the thermal energy analyzer (TEA) for trace determination of volatile and non-volatile N-nitroso compounds', *Analyt. Chem.*, *47*, 1188–91

Fisher, R.E.W. (1962) 'Lung cancer propaganda', *Brit. Med. J.*, (*i*), 802

Fishman, L. (1976) 'More rights for airplane passengers than for hospital patients. A report on smoking policies in Metropolitan Washington D.C. Hospitals', *Washington, D.C. Public Citizen's Health Research Group*, 4 April 1976, pp. 1–21

Fleig, C. (1908) 'Influence de la fumée de tabac et de la nicotine sous la développement de l'organisme', *C.R. Soc. Biol.* (Paris), *64*, 683–5

Fodor, G.G. & Winneke, G. (1972) 'Effect of low CO concentrations on resistance to monotony and on psychomotor capacity', *Staub-Reinhalt Luft*, *32*, 46–54

Folinsbee, L.J., Silverman, F. & Shephard, R.J. (1975) 'Exercise responses following ozone exposure', *J. Appl. Physiol.*, *38*, 996–1001

Fontana, V.J., Redisch, W., Nemir, R.L., Smith, M.K., Decrinis, K. & Sulzberger, M.B. (1959) 'Studies in tobacco hypersensitivity III Reactions to skin tests and peripheral vascular responses', *J. Allergy*, *30*, 241–9

Forbes, W.H., Dill, D.B., de Silva, H. & Van Deventer, F.M. (1937) 'The influence of moderate carbon monoxide poisoning upon the ability to drive automobiles', *J. Industr. Hyg. Toxicol.*, *19*, 598–603

Forbes, W.H., Sargent, F. & Roughton, F.J.W. (1945) 'The rate of carbon monoxide uptake by normal man', *Amer. J. Physiol.*, *143*, 594–608

Forgacs, J. & Carll, W.T. (1966) 'Mycotoxicoses: toxic fungi in tobaccos', *Science*, *152*, 1634–5

Foulds, W.S., Chisholm, J.A., Bronte-Stewart, J. & Wilson, T. (1969) 'Cyanide-induced optic neuropathy' in J. Francois (ed.), *Occupational and medication hazards in ophthalmology*, Karger, Basel, pp. 350–8

François, J., de Rouck, A., Cambie, E. & Zanen, A. (1974) L'electrodiagnostic des affections retiniennes (Etude des potentiels de répos et d'action retiniens)', *Bull. Soc. Belge d'Ophthalmol.*, *166*, 320–41

Frazer, W.M. & Stallybrass, C.O. (1948) *Textbook of public health*, E.S. Livingstone, Edinburgh

Frazier, T.M., Davis, G.H., Goldstein, H. & Goldberg, I.D. (1961) 'Cigarette smoking and prematurity. A prospective study', *Amer. J. Obst. Gynecol.*, *81*, 988–96

Frey, A.H. (1968) 'Electrical charge distribution and olfactory methodology and theory', *Psychol. Bull.*, *69*, 390–5

Galuskinová, A.V. (1964) '3-4 Benzpyrene determination in the smoky atmosphere of social meeting rooms and restaurants. A contribution to the problem of the noxiousness of so-called passive smoking', *Neoplasma*, *11* (5), 465–8

Garn, S.M., Hoff, K. & McCabe, K.D. (1977) 'Is there nutritional mediation of the "smoking effect" on the fetus', *Amer. J. Clin. Nutr.*, *32*, 1181–7

Garvey, D.J. & Longo, L.D. (1978) 'Chronic low level maternal carbon monoxide exposure and fetal growth and development', *Biol. Reprod.*, *19*, 8–14

Gastrin, G. & Ramstrom, L.M. (1979) 'How to reach and convince pregnant women to give up smoking' in J.L. Schwartz (ed.), *Progress in Smoking*

Cessation, Amer. Cancer Soc., New York, pp. 154–9

Gayrard, P., Orehek, J., Grimaud, C.H. & Charpin, J. (1974) 'Bronchoconstriction due à l'inhalation de fumée de tabac: effets comparés chez le sujet normal et l'asthmatique', *Bull. Physio-Path. Resp.*, *10*, 451–61

Gennser, G., Marsal, K. & Brantmark, B. (1975) 'Maternal smoking and fetal breathing movements', *Amer. J. Obst. Gynecol.*, *123*, 861–7

Gilbert, J.A.S. & Lindsey, A.J. (1957) 'The thermal decomposition of some tobacco constituents', *Brit. J. Cancer*, *11*, 398–402

Ginsberg, M.D. & Myers, R.E. (1976) 'Fetal brain injury after maternal carbon monoxide intoxication. Clinical and neuropathologic aspects', *Neurol.*, *26*, 15–23

Glasson, W.A. & Heuss, J.M. (1977) 'Synthesis and evaluation of potential atmospheric eye irritants', *Env. Sci. Technol.*, *11*, 395–8

Godin, G., Wright, G. & Shephard, R.J. (1972) 'Urban exposure to carbon monoxide', *Arch. Env. Health*, *25*, 305–13

Goldsmith, J.R. (1970) 'Contribution of motor vehicle exhaust, industry and cigarette smoking to community carbon monoxide exposures', *Ann. N.Y. Acad. Sci.*, *174*, 122–34

Goldsmith, J.R. & Aronow, W.S. (1975) 'Carbon monoxide and coronary heart disease: a review', *Environ. Res.*, *10*, 236–48

Goldstein, H. (1977) 'Smoking in pregnancy: some notes on the statistical controversy', *Brit. J. Prev. Soc. Med.*, *31*, 13

Gottier, P.L. (1979) 'No smoking in public places – the law is working', *Amer. Lung Assoc. Bull.*, *65*, 10–13

Goujard, J., Rumeau, C. & Schwartz, D. (1975) 'Smoking during pregnancy, stillbirth and abruptio placentae', *Biomedicine*, *23*, 20–2

Grayson, M. & Keates, R.H. (1969) *Manual of diseases of the cornea*, Little, Brown & Co., Boston

Green, G.M. & Carolin, D. (1967) 'The depressant effect of cigarette smoke on the in vitro antibacterial activity of alveolar macrophages', *New Engl. J. Med.*, *276*, 421–7

Green, H.L. & Lane, W.R. (1964) *Particulate clouds: dirts, smokes and mists*, Van Nostrand, Princeton, NJ

Greenberg, L.A., Lester, D. & Haggard, H.W. (1952) 'The absorption of narcotics in tobacco smoking', *J. Pharmacol. Ther.*, *109*, 162–7

Greiner, I. (1936) Nikotinvergiftung, beobachtet bei einein saeugling', *Jahrb. f. Kinderheilkunde*, *96*, 131–2

Grimmer, G., Boehnke, H. & Harke, H.P. (1977) 'Zum Problem des Passivrauchens: Aufnahme von polycyclischen aromatischen Kohlenwasserstoffen durch Einatmen von zigarettenrauchhaltiger Luft', *Int. Archiv. Occup. Env. Health*, *40*, 93–9

Gritz, E.R. & Jarvik, M.E. (1978) in *Handbook of Psychopharmacology*, Vol. II., Plenum Press, New York, pp. 426–64

Grob, K. (1962) 'Zur Gaschromatographie des Cigarettenrauches, 2. Teil: Verfeinerte Trennung mit Hilfe von Kapillarkolonnen', *Beitr. Tabakforsch.*, *1*, 315–23

Groll-Knapp, E., Wagner, H., Hanck, H. & Harder, M. (1972) 'Effects of low carbon monoxide concentrations on vigilance and computer-analyzed brain potentials', *Staub-Reinhalt Luft.*, *32*, 64–8

Grunwald, C., Davis, D.L. & Bush, L.P. (1971) 'Cholesterol in cigarette smoke condensate', *J. Agr. Food Chem.*, *19*, 138–9

Guerin, M. (1959) 'Tumeure pulmonaires et cancer buccal chez le rat soumis à l'inhalation de fumée de sigarette', *Bull. de l'Assoc. Franç. pour l'étude du Cancer*, *46*, 295–309

Guerin, M.R. (1971) 'Detection of sulfur-containing compounds in the gas phase of cigarette smoke', *Analyt. Letters*, *4* (11), 751–9

Guillan, G.|& Gy, A. (1907) 'Récherches expérimentales sur l'influence de l'intoxication tabagique sur la gestation', *C.R. Soc. Biol.* (Paris), *63*, 583–4

Guillerm, R., Badré, R., Hée, J. & Masurel, G. (1972) 'Composition de la fumée de tabac. Analyse des facteurs de nuisance', *Rev. Tuberc. Pneumol.*, *36*, 187–208

Guthrie, F.E. (1968) 'The nature and significance of pesticide residues on tobacco and in tobacco smoke', *Beitr. Tabakforsch.*, *4*, 229–46

—— (1973) 'Pending legislative restrictions on the use of agricultural chemicals on tobacco', *Beitr. zur Tabakforsch.*, *7* (3), 195–202

Haagen-Smit, A.J., Brunelle, M.F. & Hara, J. (1959) 'Nitrogen content of smokes from different types of tobacco', *A.M.A. Arch. Industr. Health*, *20*, 399–400

Haase, E. & Muller, W. (1971) 'Messbare Beeinflussung des EOG durch Zigarettenrauchen', *Klin. Monatsblatter für Augenheilkunde*, *158*, 677–81

Haberman-Brueschke, J.D., Brueschke, E.E., Isard, H.J. & Gershon-Cohen, J. (1965) 'Effect of smoking on skin temperature as demonstrated by the thermograph', *J. Albert Einstein Med. Center*, *13*, 205–10

Hackney, J.D., Kaufman, G.A., Lashier, H. & Lynn, K. (1962) 'Rebreathing estimate of carbon monoxide hemoglobin', *Arch. Environ. Health*, *5*, 300–7

Hajeri, H., Spira, A., Frydman, R. & Papiernik-Berkhuer, E. (1979) 'Smoking during pregnancy and maternal weight gain', *J. Perinatal Med.*, *7*, 33–8

Halperin, M.H., McFarland, R.A., Niven, J.I. & Roughton, F.J.W. (1959) 'The time course of the effects of carbon monoxide on visual thresholds', *J. Physiol.*, *146*, 583–93

Hamosh, P. & DaSilva, A.M.T. (1977) 'The effect on expiratory flow rates of smoking three cigarettes in rapid succession', *Chest*, *72*, 610–13

Hamosh, M., Simon, M.R. & Hamosh, P. (1979) 'Effect of nicotine on the development of fetal and suckling rats', *Biol. Neonate*, *35*, 290–7

Hansson, E. & Schmiterlow, C.G. (1962) 'Physiological disposition and fate of C^{14} labelled nicotine in mice and rats', *J. Pharm. Exp. Therap.*, *137*, 91–102

Hardy, J.B. & Mellits, E.D. (1972) 'Does maternal smoking during pregnancy have a long-term effect on the child', *Lancet*, *2*, 1332–6

Harke, H.P. (1970) 'Zum Problem des "Passiv-rauchens". I. Ueber den Einfluss des Rauchens auf die CO-Konzentration in Bueroraeumen', *Munch. Med. Wochenschr.*, *112*, 2328–34

Harke, H.P., Baars, A., Frahm, B., Peters, H. & Schultz, C. (1972) 'The problem of passive smoking. The concentration of smoke constituents in the air of large and small rooms as a function of the number of cigarettes smoked and of time', *Int. Archiv. f. Arbeitsmed.*, *29*, 323–39

Harke, H.P. & Bleichert, A. (1972) 'Zum problem des passiv-rauchens', *Int. Archiv. f. Arbeitsmed.*, *29*, 312–22

Harke, H.P., Liedl, W. & Denker, D. (1974) 'Zum Problem des Passivrauchens II. Untersuchungen Ueber den Kohlenmonoxidgehalt der Luft im Kraftfahrzeug durch das Rauchen von Zigaretten', *Int. Archiv. f. Arbeitsmed.*, *33*, 207–20

Harke, H.P. & Peters, H. (1974) 'Zum Problem des Passivrauchens III. Ueber den Einfluss des Rauchens auf die CO-Konzentration im Kraftfahrzeug bei Fahrten im Stadtgebiet', *Int. Archiv. f. Arbeitsmed.*, *33*, 221–9

Harlap, S. & Davies, A.M. (1974) 'Infant admissions to hospital and maternal smoking', *Lancet*, (*i*), (7857) 529–32 |

Harmsen, E. & Effenberger, E. (1957) 'Tobacco smoke in transportation vehicles, living and working rooms', *Archiv. f. Hyg. u. Bakteriol.*, *141*, 383–400

Harris, J.E. (1979) *Smoking during pregnancy. Preliminary results from the National Clearing House on Smoking and Health, 1975 Prevalence data* (cited by Surgeon General, 1979)

Harris, R.J.C. & Negroni, G. (1967) 'Production of lung carcinomas in C57BL mice exposed to cigarette smoke and air mixture', *Brit. Med. J.*, *4* (5580), 637–41

Harrison, K.L. & McKenna, H. (1977) 'The effect of maternal smoking on cord blood erythrocytes', *Austr. N.Z. J. Obst. Gynecol.*, *17*, 160–2

Harvaky, J. (1939) 'Tobacco skin reactions and their clinical significance', *J. Invest. Dermatol.*, *2*, 257–79

Harvey, E.B., Dettmers, M.V. & Marsden, L.R. (1974) 'The air we perceive. A study of attitudes towards air pollution in Toronto for the York–Toronto Lung Association', unpublished report, York–Toronto Lung Association, Willowdale

Hatcher, R.A. & Crosby, K. (1927) 'The elimination of nicotine in the milk', *J. Pharm. Exp. Therap.*, *32*, 1–6

Haworth, J.C. & Ford, J.D. (1972) 'Comparison of the effects of maternal undernutrition and exposure to cigarette smoke on the cellular growth of the rat fetus', *Amer. J. Obstet. Gynecol.*, *112*, 653–6

Hecht, S.S., Ornaf, R.M. & Hoffmann, D. (1975) 'Chemical studies on tobacco smoke. XXXIII. N'-nitrosonornicotine in tobacco: analysis of possible contributing factors and biologic implications', *J. Nat. Cancer Inst.*, *54* (5), 1237–44

Heinonen, O.P., Sloane, D. & Shapiro, S. (1977) *Birth defects and drugs in pregnancy*, Publishing Sciences Group, Acton, Mass.

Hellman, L.M., Johnson, H.L., Tolles, W.E. & Jones, E.H. (1961) 'Some factors affecting the fetal heart rate', *Amer. J. Obstet. Gynecol.*, *82*, 1055–63

Hellman, L.M. & Pritchard, J.A. (1971) *Williams Obstetrics*, 14th edn, Appleton–Century–Crofts, New York

Henderson, M. & Apthorp, G.H. (1960) 'Rapid method for the estimation of carbon monoxide in blood', *Brit. Med. J.*, (*ii*), 1853–4

Hengen, N. & Hengen, M. (1978) 'Gas-liquid chromatographic determination of nicotine and cotinine in plasma', *Clin. Chem.*, *24*, 50–3

Hengy, H. & Thirion, J. (1970) 'The determination of Malathion residues in tobacco smoke condensate', *Beitr. Tabakforsch.*, *5*, 175–8

Henry, F.M. & Fitzhenry, J.R. (1950) 'Oxygen metabolism of moderate exercise, with some observations on effects of tobacco smoking', *J. Appl. Physiol.*, *2*, 464–8

Hernandez, J.A., Anderson, A.E., Holmes, W.L. & Foraker, A.G. (1966) 'Pulmonary parenchymal defects in dogs following prolonged cigarette smoke exposure', *Amer. Rev. Resp. Dis.*, *93*, 78–83

Heron, H.J. (1962) 'The effect of smoking during pregnancy. A review with a preview', *New Z. Med. J.*, *61*, 545–8

Herriot, A., Billewicz, Z. & Hytten, F.E. (1962) 'Cigarette smoking in pregnancy', *Lancet*, (*i*), 771–3

Herrmann, K. (1964) 'Über die phenolischen Inhaltsstoffe des Tabaks und des Tabakrauches', *Beitr. Tabakforsch.*, *2*, 159–79

Herxheimer, A., Griffiths, R.L., Hamilton, B. & Wakefield, M. (1967) 'Circulatory effects of nicotine aerosol inhalations and cigarette smoking in man', *Lancet*, (*ii*), 754–5

Hess, H.A. (1971) 'A contribution to the problem of passive smoking', *Munch. Med. Wschr.*, *113*, 705–6

Hexter, A.C. & Goldsmith, J.R. (1971) 'Carbon monoxide: association of community air pollution with mortality', *Science*, *172*, 265–7

Hill, E.P., Hill, J.R., Power, G.G. & Longo, L.D. (1977) 'Carbon monoxide exchanges between the human fetus and mother: a mathematical model',

Amer. J. Physiol., *232*, H311–23

Hill, P. & Marquardt, H. (1980) 'Plasma and urine changes after smoking different brands of cigarettes', *Clin. Pharm. Therap.*, *27*, 652–8

Himmelberger, D.U., Brown, B.W. & Cohen, E.N. (1978) 'Cigarette smoking during pregnancy and the occurrence of spontaneous abortion and congenital abnormality', *Amer. J. Epidemiol.*, *108*, 470–9

Hinds, W.C. & First, M.W. (1975) 'Concentrations of nicotine and tobacco smoke in public places', *New Engl. J. Med.*, *292*, 844–5

Hirayama, T. (1981) 'Non-smoking wives of heavy smokers have a higher risk of lung cancer: a study from Japan', *Brit. Med. J.*, *282*, 183–5

Hobbs, M.E. (1957) 'Chemical equilibria in the gas phase of cigaret smoke', *Tobacco Sci.*, *1*, 74–7

Hoegg, U.R. (1972) 'Cigarette smoke in closed spaces', *Environ. Health Perspect.*, *2*, 117–28

Hoffmann, D., Rathkamp, G. & Wynder, E.L. (1963) 'Comparison of the yields of several selected components in the smoke from different products', *J. Nat. Cancer Inst.*, *31*, 627–37

Hoffmann, D., Schmeltz, I., Hecht, S.S. & Wynder, E.L. (1976) 'Chemical studies on tobacco smoke XXXIX. On the identification of carcinogens, tumor promoters and co-carcinogens in tobacco smoke in E.L. Wynder, D. Hoffmann & G.B. Gori (eds.), *Proceedings of the Third World Conference on Smoking and Health, New York, June 2–5, 1975. Vol. 1. Modifying the risk for the smoker*, National Cancer Institute, Bethesda, Md., DHEW Publication 76, 1221, pp. 125–45

Hoffmann, D. & Wynder, E.L. (1972) 'Smoke of cigarettes and little cigars: an analytical comparison', *Science*, *178*, 1197–9

Holland, R.H., Kozlowski, E.J. & Booker, L. (1963) 'The effect of cigarette smoke on the respiratory system of the rabbit. A final report', *Cancer*, *16*, 612–15

Hollingsworth, D.R., Moser, R.J., Carlson, J.W. & Thompson, K.T. (1976) 'Abnormal adolescent primiparous pregnancy: association of race, human chorionic somatomammotropin production and smoking', *Amer. J. Obstetr. Gynecol.*, *126*, 230–7

Horning, E.C., Horning, M.G., Carroll, D.J., Stillwell, R.N. & Dzidic, I. (1973) 'Nicotine in smokers, non-smokers and room air', *Life Sci.*, *13*, 1331–46

Horton, A.D. & Guerin, M.R. (1974) 'Quantitative determination of sulfur compounds in the gas phase of cigarette smoke', *J. Chromat.*, *90*, 63–70

Horvath, S.M. (1973) in *Proceedings of conference of health effects of air pollutants. Assembly of Life Sciences NAS-NRC*, Committee on Public Works, US Senate, Serial #93–15, pp. 127–39

Horvath, S.M., Dahms, T.E. & O'Hanlon, J.F. (1971) 'Carbon monoxide and human vigilance – a deleterious effect of present urban concentrations', *Arch. Environ. Health*, *23*, 343–7

Horvath, S.M., Raven, P.B., Dahms, T.E. & Gray, D.J. (1975) 'Maximal aerobic capacity at different levels of carboxyhemoglobin', *J. Appl. Physiol.*, *38*, 300–3

Hrubes, V. & Baettig, K. (1970) 'Effects of inhaled cigarette smoke on swimming endurance in the rat', *Arch. Env. Health*, *21*, 20–4

Hudson, D.B., Meisami, E. & Timiras, P.S. (1973) 'Brain development in offspring of rats treated with nicotine during pregnancy', *Experientia*, *29*, 286–8

Hudson, G.S. & Rucker, M.P. (1945) 'Spontaneous abortion', *J. Amer. Med. Assoc.*, *129*, 542

International Committee (1974) 'Machine smoking of cigars', *Coresta Information Bulletin 1974*, (*1*), 31–4

Irving, D.W. & Yamomoto, T. (1963) 'Cigarette smoking and cardiac output', *Brit. Heart J.*, *25*, 126–32

James, G. (1964) 'Health challenges today', *Amer. Rev. Resp. Dis.*, *90*, 349–58

Jarboe, C.H. & Rosene, C.J. (1961) 'Volatile products of pyrolysis of nicotine', *J. Chem. Soc. 1961*, 2455–8

Jarvinen, P.A. & Osterlund, K. (1963) 'Effect of smoking during pregnancy on the fetus, placenta and delivery', *Ann. Pediatr. Fenn.*, *9*, 18–26

Jayle, G.E., Metge, P., Chaix, A., Vola, J.L. & Tassy, A. (1972) 'Exploration functionnelle des Neurites Optiques Alcoolo-Tabagiques', *Arch. d'Ophthalmol.*, *32*, Suppl. 1, 79–86

Jermini, C., Weber, A. & Grandjean, E. (1976) 'Quantitative Bestimmung verschiedener Gasphasen Komponenten des Nebenstromrauches von Zigaretten in der Raumluft als Beitrag zum Problem des Passiv-rauchens', *Int. Arch. Occup. Environ. Hlth.*, *36*, 169–81

Johannson, C.R. (1976) 'Tobacco smoke in room air – an experimental investigation of odour perception and irritating effects', *Building Services Engineer*, *43*, 254–62

Johannson, C.R. & Ronge, H. (1965) 'Akuta irritationseffekter av tobaksrök i rumsluft', *Nord. Hyg. Tidskr.*, *46*, 45–50

―――― (1966) 'Klimatinverkan på lukt och irritationseffeki av tobaksrök. Preliminärt meddelande', *Nord. Hyg. Tidskr.*, *47*, 33–9

Johnson, W.R., Hale, R.W., Nedlock, J.W., Grubbs, H.J. & Powell, D.H. (1973a) 'The distribution of products between mainstream and sidestream smoke', *Tobacco Sci.*, *17*, 141–4

Johnson, W.R., Hale, R.W., Clough, S.C. & Chen, P.H. (1973b) 'Chemistry of the conversion of nitrate nitrogen to smoke products', *Nature*, *243*, 223–5

Johnstone, R.A.W. & Plimmer, J.R. (1959) 'The chemical constituents of tobacco and tobacco smoke', *Chem. Rev.*, *59*, 885–936

Jones, R.H., Ellicott, M.F., Cadigan, J.B. & Gaensler, E.A. (1958) 'The relationship between alveolar and blood carbon monoxide concentrations during breath holding', *J. Lab. Clin. Med.*, *51*, 553–64

Jones, R.M. & Fagan, R. (1974) 'Application of mathematical model for the building of carbon monoxide from cigarette smoking in rooms and houses', *Amer. Soc. Heat. Refrig. Air Cond. Eng. Journal* (August 1974), 49–53

Joyner, R.E. (1964) 'Effect of cigarette smoking on olfactory acuity', *Arch. Otolaryngol.*, *80*, 576–9

Juchan, M.R. (1971) 'Human placental hydroxylation of 3–4 benzpyrene during early gestation and at term', *Toxicol. Appl. Pharmacol.*, *18*, 665–75

Justus, D.E. & Adams, D.A. (1976) 'Evaluation of tobacco hypersensitivity responses in the mouse. A potential animal model for critical study of tobacco allergy', *Internat. Arch. Allergy Appl. Immunol.*, *51*, 687–95

Kagan, A., Harris, B.R., Winkelstein, W., Jonson, K.G., Kato, H., Syme, S.L., Rhoods, G.G., Gay, M.L., Nichaman, M.Z., Hamilton, H.B. & Tillotson, J. (1974) 'Epidemiologic studies of coronary heart disease and stroke in Japanese men living in Japan, Hawaii and California: Demographic, physical, dietary and biochemical characteristics', *J. Chron. Dis.*, *27*, 345–64

Keith, C.H. (1972) 'Modification of tobacco smoke' in I. Schmeltz (ed.), *The chemistry of tobacco and tobacco smoke*, Plenum Press, New York, pp. 149–66

Keith, C.H. & Derrick, J.C. (1960) 'Measurement of the particle size distribution and concentration of cigarette smoke by the "conifuge"', *J. Colloid Sci.*, *15*, 340–56

Keith, C.H. & Tesh, P.G. (1965) *Tobacco Sci.*, *9*, 61–4

Kensler, C.J. (1960) 'Components of pharmacological interest in cigarette smoke',

Ann. N.Y. Acad. Sci., *90*, 43-7

Kerka, W.F. & Humphreys, C.M. (1956) 'Temperature and humidity effects on odor perception', *ASHAE Trans.*, *62*, 531-52

Kiefer, J.E. (1972) 'Filtration of cigarette smoke' in I. Schmeltz (ed.), *The chemistry of tobacco and tobacco smoke*, Plenum Press, New York, pp. 167-76

Kittel, G. (1976) 'Results of clinical olfactometric studies', *Rhinology*, *14*, 99-108

Kjeldsen, K., Astrup, P. & Wanstrup, J. (1972) 'Ultrastructural intimal changes in the rabbit aorta after a moderate carbon monoxide exposure', *Atherosclerosis*, *16*, 67-82

Kline, J., Stein, Z.A., Susser, M. & Warburton, D. (1977) 'Smoking: a risk factor for spontaneous abortion', *New Engl. J. Med.*, *297*, 793-6

Knudson, R.J., Lebowitz, M.D., Burton, A.P. & Knudson, D.E. (1977) 'The closing volume test: evaluation of nitrogen and bolus methods in a random population', *Amer. Rev. Resp. Dis.*, *115*, 423-34

Kreis, B., Peltier, A., Fournand, S. & Dupin-Girod, S. (1970) 'Reaction de precipitation entre certains serums humains et des extraits soluble de tabac', *Ann. Med. Interne.*, *121*, 437-40

Krippner, R.A. & Heimstra, N.W. (1969) 'Effects of smoking on peripheral visual acuity', unpublished report, Dept. of Psychology, University of South Dakota, Vermilion, S. Dakota, pp. 1-57

Kuhn, H.A. (1966) 'A comparative study of cigarette and cigar smoke' in *Proceedings of 4th International Tobacco Scientific Congress*, National Tobacco Board, Greece, pp. 967-71

Kullander, S. & Kaellen, B. (1971) 'A prospective study of smoking and pregnancy', *Acta Obst. Gynecol. Scand.*, *50*, 83-94

Kuller, L.H., Radford, E.P., Swift, D., Perper, J.A. & Fisher, R. (1975) 'Carbon monoxide and heart attacks', *Arch. Environ. Health*, *30*, 477-82

Kurt, T.L., Mogielnicki, R.P. & Chandler, J.E. (1978) 'Association of the frequency of acute cardio-respiratory complaints with ambient levels of carbon monoxide', *Chest*, *74*, 10-14

Lambert, B., Lindblad, A., Nordenskyjold, M. & Werelius, B. (1978) 'Increased frequency of sister chromatid exchanges in cigarette smokers', *Hereditas*, *88*, 147-9

Lancet (1979) 'Smoking and intra-interine growth' (editorial), *Lancet*, (*i*), 536-7

Landesman-Dwyer, S. & Emmanuel, I. (1979) 'Smoking during pregnancy', *Teratology*, *19*, 119-25

Landesman-Dwyer, S., Killer, L.S. & Streissguth, A.P. (1978) 'Naturalistic observations of newborns: effects of maternal alcohol intake', *Alcoholism Clin. Exp. Res.*, *2*, 171-7

Landmann, H. (1976) 'Empfehlungen zur Pravention von Tabakschaden' in *Gesundheitsschaden durch Rauchen − Moglichkeiten einer Prophylaxe*, Akademie-Verlag, Berlin, pp. 195-201

Langford, E.R., Thompson, E. & Tripp, S.C. (1980) 'Smoking and health education during pregnancy: evaluation of a program for women in pre-natal classes', unpublished report, Dept. of Health Administration, University of Toronto, Toronto

Larson, P.S. & Silvette, H. (1969) *Tobacco: experimental and clinical studies. A comprehensive account of world literature. Supplement*, Williams & Wilkins, Baltimore, pp. 153-98

Lauwerys, R., Buchet, J.P., Roels, H. & Hubermont, G. (1978) 'Placental transfer of lead, mercury, cadmium and carbon monoxide in women. 1. Comparison of the distribution of the biological indices in maternal and umbilical cord blood', *Env. Res.*, *15*, 278-89

Lawther, P.J. & Commins, B.T. (1970) 'Cigarette smoking and exposure to carbon monoxide', *Ann. N.Y. Acad. Sci.*, *174*, 135-47

Lebowitz, M.D. & Burrows, B. (1976) 'Respiratory symptoms related to smoking habits of family adults', *Chest*, *69*, 48-50

Leeder, S.R., Corkhill, R., Irwig, L.M., Holland, W.W. & Colley, J.R.T. (1976) 'Influence of family factors on the incidence of lower respiratory illness during the first year of life', *Brit. J. Prev. Soc. Med.*, *30*, 203-12

Lehtovirta, P. & Forss, M. (1978) 'The acute effect of smoking on intervillous blood flow of the placenta', *Brit. J. Obstet. Gyn.*, *85*, 729-31

Lemp, M.A., Dohlman, C.H. & Kuwabara, T. (1971) 'Dry eye secondary to mucus deficiency', *Trans. Amer. Acad. Ophthalmol. & Otol.*, *75*, 1223-7

Lemp, M.A. & Hamill, J.R. (1973) 'Factors affecting tear film breakup in normal eyes', *Arch. Ophthalmol.*, *89*, 103-5

Leuchtenberger, C., Leuchtenberger, R., Zebrun, W. & Shaffer, P. (1960a) 'A correlated histological, cytological and cytochemical study of the tracheobronchial tree and lungs of mice exposed to cigarette smoke. II. Varying responses of major bronchi to cigarette smoke, absence of bronchogenic carcinoma after prolonged exposure and disappearance of bronchial lesions after cessation of exposure', *Cancer*, *13*, 721-32

Leuchtenberger, R., Leuchtenberger, C., Zebrun, W. & Shaffer, P. (1960b) 'A correlated histological, cytological and cytochemical study of the tracheobronchial tree and lungs of mice exposed to cigarette smoke. III. Unaltered incidence of grossly visible adenomatous lung tumours in female CF mice after prolonged exposure to cigarette smoke', *Cancer*, *13*, 956-8

L'Heureux, R. (1979) 'L'usage du tabac dans les endroits publics et la protection des non-fumeurs', *President, Consil Consultatif de l'Environnement*, Gouvernement du Québec, Québec, Canada

Lightfoot, N.F. (1972) 'Chronic carbon monoxide exposure', *Proc. Roy. Soc. Med.*, *65*, 16-17

Lilienthal, J.L., Riley, R.L., Prommel, D.D. & Franke, R.E. (1946) 'The relationships between carbon monoxide, oxygen and hemoglobin in the blood of man at altitude', *Amer. J. Physiol.*, *145*, 351-8

Lima, A.O. & Rocha, G. (1949) 'Cutaneous reactions to tobacco antigen in allergic and non-allergic children', *Ann. Allergy*, 7, 528-31

Lipp, G. (1965) 'Zur definition der selektivitat und der verscheidenen rauchstrome der cigarette', *Beitr. Tabakforsch.*, *3*, 220-2

Loehr, J., Ardelt, W. & Dehnhard, F. (1972) 'Nikotinarteriopathie der plazenta', *Geburtshilfe und Frauenheilkunde*, *32*, 932-4

Long, P.H. (1964) 'The problem of smoking', *Medical Times*, *92*, 411-12

Longo, L.D. (1970) 'Carbon monoxide in the pregnant mother and fetus and its exchange across the placenta', *Ann. N.Y. Acad. Sci.*, *174*, 313-41

—— (1972) 'Disorders of placental transfer' in N.S. Assali & C.R. Brinkman (eds.), *Pathophysiology of gestation*, Academic Press, New York, pp. 1-76

—— (1977) 'The biological effects of carbon monoxide on the pregnant woman, fetus and newborn infant', *Amer. J. Obstet. Gynecol.*, *129*, 69-103

Longo, L.D. & Hill, E.P. (1977) 'Carbon monoxide uptake and elimination in fetal and maternal sheep', *Amer. J. Physiol.*, *232*, H324-30

Longo, L.D., Wyatt, J.F., Hewitt, C.W. & Gilbert, R.D. (1978) 'A comparison of circulatory responses to hypoxic hypoxia and carbon monoxide hypoxia in fetal blood flow and oxygenation' in L.D. Longo & D.D. Reneau (eds.), *Fetal and newborn cardiovascular physiology: fetal and newborn circulation Vol. 2*, Garland STPM Press, New York, pp. 259-87

Lorenz, E., Stewart, H.L., Daniel, J.H. & Nelson, C.V. (1943) 'The effects of breathing tobacco smoke on Strain A mice', *Cancer Research*, *3*, 123

Lowe, C.R. (1959) 'Effect of mothers' smoking habits on birthweight of their children', *Brit. Med. J.*, *2*, 673-6

Luquette,A.J., Landiss, C.W. & Merki, D.J. (1970) 'Some immediate effects of a smoking environment on children of elementary school age', *J. Sch. Health*, *40*, 533-6

Maas, A.H.J., Hamelink, M.L. & de Leeuw, R.J.M. (1970) 'An evaluation of the spectrophotometric determination of HbO_2, HbCO and Hb in blood with the CO-oximeter IL 182', *Clin. Chim. Acta*, *29*, 303-10

McDermott, M.G. (1962) 'Acute respiratory effects of the inhalation of coal dust particles', *J. Physiol.*, *162*, 53p

McFarland, R.A. (1973) 'Low level exposure to carbon monoxide and driving performance', *Arch. Environ. Health*, *28*, 355-9

McFarland, R.A., Roughton, F.J.W., Halperin, M.H. & Niven, J.J. (1944) 'The effects of carbon monoxide and altitude on visual thresholds', *J. Aviat. Med.*, *15*, 381-94

McGarry, J.M. & Andrews, J. (1972) 'Smoking in pregnancy and vitamin B_{12} metabolism', *Brit. Med. J.*, *2*, 74-7

McIlvaine, P.M., Nelson, W.C. & Bartlett, D. (1969) 'Temporal variation of carboxyhemoglobin concentrations', *Arch. Env. Health*, *19*, 83-91

MacMahon, B., Alpert, M. & Salber, E.J. (1966) 'Infant weight and parental smoking habits', *Amer. J. Epidemiol.*, *82*, 247-65

McNall, P.E. (1975) 'Practical methods of reducing airborne contaminants in interior spaces', *Arch. Env. Health*, *30*, 552-6

McRae, B.C. & Choi-Lao, A.T.H. (1978) 'National survey on smoking and health education in pre-natal classes in Canada', *Canad. J. Publ. Health*, *69*, 427-30

Magee, P.N. & Barnes, J.M. (1966) 'Carcinogenic nitroso compounds', *Adv. Cancer Res.*, *10*, 163-246

Malcolm, S. & Shephard, R.J. (1978) 'Personality and sexual behavior of the adolescent smoker', *Amer. J. Drug Alcohol Abuse*, *5*, 87-96

Manning, F.A. & Feyerabend, C. (1976) 'Cigarette smoking and fetal breathing movements', *Brit. J. Obstetr. Gynec.*, *83*, 262-70

Martin, J.C. & Becker, R.F. (1971) 'The effects of maternal nicotine absorption or hypoxic episodes upon appetitive behavior of rat offspring', *Dev. Psychobiol.*, *4*, 133-47

Martin, R.R., Lindsey, D., Despas, P., Bruce, D., Leroux, M., Anthonisen, N.R. & Macklem, P.T. (1975) 'The early detection of airway obstruction', *Amer. Rev. Resp. Dis.*, *111*, 119-25

Masuda, Y. & Hoffmann, D. (1969) 'Quantitative determination of 1 naphthylamine and 2 naphthylamine in cigarette smoke', *Anal. Chem.*, *41*, 650-2

Mattina, C.F. & Selke, W.A. (1975) 'Reconstituted tobacco sheets' in E.L. Wynder, D. Hoffmann & G.B. Gori (eds.), *Proceedings of the Third World Conference on Smoking and Health*, National Cancer Institute, Bethesda, Md., *DHEW Publication*, *76*, 1221, pp. 67-72

Matzker, J. (1965) 'Reichen und Lebensalter − Reichen und Rauchen', *Unschau*, *21*, 673

Mau, G. & Netter, P. (1974) 'The effects of paternal smoking on perinatal mortality and the incidence of malformation' ('Die Auswirkungen des viaterlichen Zigarettenkongums auf die perinatale Sterblichkiet und die Missbildungshaufigkeit'), *Dtsch. Med. Wschr.*, *99*, 1113-18

Maugh, T.H. (1972) 'Carbon monoxide: natural sources dwarf man's output', *Science*, *177*, 338-9

Maxwell, J. (1962) 'Cigarette smoking and lung cancer', *Brit. Med. J.*, *(i)*, 872-3

Medical Tribune (1978) 'MDs who gave up smoking allow it in waiting rooms', *Medical Tribune, 19*, 1, 7

Medizinische Monatschrift (1975) 'Rauchverbot bei Fortibildungsveranstaltungen', *Medizinische Monatschrift, 29*, 141-2

Medizinische-Welt (1978) 'Dauerstreit: Rauchen', *Medizinische Welt, 29*, 25-6

Mehra, K.S., Roy, P.N. & Khare, B.B. (1976) 'Tobacco smoking and glaucoma', *Ann. Ophthalmol., 8*, 462-4

Meredith, H.V. (1975) 'Relation between tobacco smoking of pregnant women and body size of their progeny: a compilation of published studies', *Human Biol., 47*, 451-72

Mertens, D.J., Kavanagh, T. & Shephard, R.J. (1978) 'Exercise rehabilitation for chronic obstructive lung disease', *Respiration, 35*, 95-107

Meyer, M.B. (1977) 'Effects of maternal smoking and altitude on birth weight and gestation' in D.M. Reed & F.J. Stanley (eds.), *The epidemiology of prematurity*, Urban & Schwarzenberg, Baltimore, pp. 81-101

—— (1978) 'How does maternal smoking affect birth weight and maternal weight gain? Evidence from the Ontario Perinatal Mortality Study', *Amer. J. Obstetr. Gynecol., 131*, 888-93

Meyer, M.B. & Comstock, G.W. (1972) 'Maternal cigarette smoking and perinatal mortality', *Amer. J. Epidemiol., 96*, 1-10

Meyer, M.B., Jonas, B.S. & Tonascia, J.A. (1976) 'Perinatal events associated with maternal smoking during pregnancy', *Amer. J. Epidemiol., 103*, 464-76

Meyer, M.B. & Tonascia, J.A. (1977) 'Maternal smoking, pregnancy complications and perinatal mortality', *Amer. J. Obstetr. Gynecol., 128*, 494-502

Meyer, M.B., Tonascia, J.A. & Buck, C. (1975) 'The inter-relationship of maternal smoking and increased perinatal mortality with other risk factors. Further analysis of the Ontario Perinatal Mortality Study 1960-61', *Amer. J. Epidemiol., 100*, 443-52

Michigan State Department of Education (1971) *The age of majority – 18: guidelines for local districts*, Michigan State Dept. of Education, Lansing, July 1971, pp. 1-20

Mikulka, P., O'Donnell, R., Jeinig, P. & Theodore, J. (1970) 'The effect of carbon monoxide on human performance', *Ann. N.Y. Acad. Sci., 174*, 409-20

Miller, F., Freeman, W.J. & Stedman, R.J. (1968) 'Effect of additives on the combustion temperature of cigarets', *Beitr. Tabakforsch., 4*, 269-74

Miller, G.H. (1978) 'The Pennsylvania Study on Passive Smoking', *J. Breathing, 41*, 5-9

Miller, H.C. & Hassanein, K. (1964) 'Maternal smoking and fetal growth of full term infants', *Pediatr. Research, 8*, 960-3

Miller, H.C., Hassanein, K. & Hensleigh, P.A. (1976) 'Fetal growth retardation in relation to maternal smoking and weight gain in pregnancy', *Amer. J. Obstetr. Gynecol., 125*, 55-60

Mitchell, R.I. (1962) 'Controlled measurement of smoke-particle retention in the respiratory tract', *Amer. Rev. Resp. Dis., 85*, 526-33

Mohr, U. & Althoff, J. (1971) 'Carcinogenic activity of aliphatic nitrosamines via the mother's milk in the offspring of Syrian Golden hamsters', *Proc. Soc. Exp. Biol. Med., 136*, 1007-9

Montgomery, M.R. & Rubin, R.J. (1971) 'The effect of carbon monoxide inhalation in "in vivo" drug metabolism in the rat', *J. Pharmacol. Exp. Therap., 179*, 465-73

Morgan, R.W. & Drance, S.M. (1975) 'Chronic open-angle glaucoma and ocular hypertension', *Brit. J. Ophthalmol., 59*, 211-15

Moser, M. (1972) 'Zur Messung der Nasenfunktion – Klinische Olfaktometrie', *Med. Monatschrift., 26*, 267-9

References 179

Moshey, R.J. (1967) 'Reconstituted tobacco sheet' in E.L. Wynder & D. Hoffmann
(eds.), *Tobacco & Tobacco Smoke*, Academic Press, New York, pp. 47–83
Mosier, H.D. & Jansons, R.A. (1973) 'Distribution and fate of nicotine in the rat
fetus', *Teratology*, *6*, 303–12
Mühlbock, O. (1955) 'Carcinogene Werking van Sigarettenrook bij Muizen', *Ned.
Tidjschrift v. Geneeskunde*, *99*, 2276–8
Mulcahy, R., Murphy, J. & Martin, F. (1970) 'Placental changes and maternal
weight in smoking and non-smoking mothers', *Amer. J. Obstetr. Gynecol.*,
106, 703–4
Mumpower, R.C., Lewis, J.S. & Touey, G.P. (1962) 'Determination of carbon
monoxide in cigarette smoke by gas chromatography', *Tobacco Sci.*, *6*, 142–5
Murphy, J. & Mulcahy, R. (1978) 'Cigarette smoking and spontaneous abortion',
Brit. Med. J., *(i)*, 988
Nadel, J.A. & Comroe, J.H. (1961) 'Acute effects of inhalation of cigarette smoke
on airway conductance', *J. Appl. Physiol.*, *16*, 713–16
Naeye, R.L. (1978a) 'Relationship of cigarette smoking to congenital
abnormalities and perinatal death', *Amer. J. Pathol.*, *90*, 289–94
—— (1978b) 'Effects of maternal cigarette smoking on the fetus and placenta',
Brit. J. Obstetr. Gynecol., *85*, 732–7
—— (1979) 'Data from US Collaborative Perinatal Project', reported to Amer.
Heart Assoc. Annual Science Writers' Forum, Hilton Head Island, S.C.,
15 January 1979
Naeye, R.L., Herkness, W.L. & Utts, J. (1977) 'Abruptio placentae and perinatal
death: a prospective study', *Amer. J. Obstetr. Gynecol.*, *128*, 740–6
Naeye, R.L., Ladis, B. & Drage, J.S. (1976) 'Sudden infant death syndrome: a
prospective study', *Amer. J. Dis. Child.*, *130*, 1207–10
Nakajima, T., Hattori, S., Tateisui, R. & Horai, T. (1972) 'Morphological changes
in the bronchial alveolar system of mice following continuous exposure to low
concentrations of nitrogen dioxide and carbon monoxide', *J. Jap. Soc. Chest
Dis.*, *10*, 16–22
National Cancer Institute (1977) *Towards less hazardous cigarettes. Report No. 3*,
National Cancer Institute, Bethesda, Md., *DHEW Publication 77–1280*,
pp. 1–152
National Clearing House for Smoking and Health (1976) *State Legislation on
Smoking and Health, 1976*, US Dept. of Health Education and Welfare, Public
Health Service Center for Disease Control 1976, pp. 1–73
—— (1977) *State Legislation on Smoking and Health, 1977*, US Dept. of
Health, Education and Welfare, Public Health Service Center for Disease
Control, *DHEW Publication CDC 78–8331*, pp. 1–79
Neuberger, M.B. (1963) *Smoke screen: tobacco and the public welfare*, Prentice
Hall, Englewood Cliffs, NJ
Neurath, G. (1969) 'Stickstoffverbindungen des Tabakrauches', *Beitr.
Tabakforsch.*, *5*, 115–33
—— (1972) 'Recent advances in knowledge of the chemical composition of
tobacco smoke' in I. Schmeltz (ed.), *The chemistry of tobacco and tobacco
smoke*, Plenum Press, New York, pp. 77–9
Neurath, G. Dünger, M., Gewe, J., Lüttich, W. & Wichern, H. (1966a)
'Untersuchungen der flüchtigen Basen des Tabakrauches', *Beitr. Tabakforsch.*,
3, 563–9
Neurath, G. & Ehmke, H. (1964) 'Examination of nitrate contents of tobacco',
Beitr. Tabakforsch., *2*, 333–44
Neurath, G., Ehmke, H. & Horstmann, H. (1964) 'Einfluss des
Feuchtigkeitsgehaltes von Cigaretten auf die Zusammensetzung des Rauches
III', *Beitr. Tabakforsch.*, *2*, 361–9

Neurath, G., Ehmke, H. & Schneemann, H. (1966b) *Beitr. Tabakforsch.*, *3*, 351

Neutel, C.L. & Buck, C. (1971) 'Effect of smoking during pregnancy on the risk of cancer in children', *J. Nat. Cancer Inst.*, *47*, 59–63

Newby, D.W., Roberts, R.J. & Bhatnagar, R.K. (1978) 'Carbon monoxide-hypoxia induced effects on catecholamines in the mature and developing rat brain', *J. Pharm. Exp. Therap.*, *206*, 61–8

Newsome, J.R. & Keith, C.H. (1965) 'Variation of the gas phase composition within a burning cigarette', *Tobacco Sci.*, *9*, 65–9

Niinimaa, V., Cole, P., Mintz, S. & Shephard, R.J. (1979) 'A head-out body plethysmograph', *J. Appl. Physiol.*, *47*, 1336–9

――― (1980) 'The switching point from nasal to oronasal breathing', *Resf. Physiol.*, *42*, 61–71

Nikonova, T.V. (1977) 'Transplacental action of benzo (α) pyrene and pyrene', *Bull. Exp. Biol. Med.*, *84*, 1025–7

Norman, V. & Keith, C.H. (1965) 'Nitrogen oxides in tobacco smoke', *Nature*, *205*, 915–16

Norman-Taylor, N. & Dickinson, V.A. (1977) 'Dangers for children in smoking families', *Community Med.*, *128*, 32–3

Oasis (1978) 'Should SSA ban smoking? 20,000 express their views', *Oasis 24* (9), 26 (US Social Security Admin.)

Obe, G. & Herha, J. (1978) 'Chromosomal aberrations in heavy smokers', *Human Genetics*, *41*, 259–63

Oberst, F.W. (1961) 'Factors affecting inhalation and retention of toxic vapors' in C.N. Davies (ed.), *Inhaled particles and vapours*, Pergamon Press, Oxford, pp. 249–66

O'Connell, C. & Logan, G. (1974) 'Parental smoking in childhood asthma', *Ann. Allergy*, *32*, 142–5

O'Donnell, R.D., Mikulka, P., Heinigs, P. & Theodore, J. (1970) 'Effects of short-term low-level carbon monoxide exposure on human performance', *US Aerospace Medical Research Laboratory Report* AMRL-TR-70–37

――― (1971) 'Low level carbon monoxide exposure and human psychomotor performance', *Toxicol. Appl. Pharmacol.*, *18*, 593–602

O'Lane, J.M. (1963) 'Some fetal effects of maternal cigarette smoking', *Obstetr. Gynecol.*, *22*, 181–4

Ontario Ministry of Health (1976) *Guidelines for the establishment of non-smoking areas*, Ministry of Health, Ontario, 76–2765, pp. 1–8

Oregon State Board of Education (1972) *Minimum standards for student conduct and discipline, including suggested guidelines and model codes*, Oregon Administrative Rules 21–050–21–085, Oregon State Board of Education, Salem

Osborne, J.S., Adamek, S. & Hobbs, M.E. (1956) 'Some components of gas phase of cigarette smoke', *Anal. Chem.*, *28*, 211–15

Osman, S. & Barson, J. (1964) 'Hydrocarbons of cigar smoke', *Tobacco*, *159*, 30–2

Osman, S., Schmeltz, I., Higman, H.C. & Stedman, R.L. (1963) 'Volatile phenols of cigar smoke', *Tobacco*, *157*, 30–2

Otto, D.A., Benignus, V.A. & Prah, J.D. (1979) 'Carbon monoxide and human time discrimination: failure to replicate Beard–Wertheim experiment', *Aviat. Space Env. Med.*, *50*, 40–3

Otto, H. (1963) 'Experimentelle Untersuchungen an Mäusen mit passiver Zigarettenrauchbeatmung', *Frankfurther Zeit. f. Pathol.*, *73*, 10–23

Owen, W.C. & Reynolds, M.L. (1967) 'The diffusion of gases through cigaret paper during smoking', *Tobacco Sci.*, *11*, 14–20

Oxhøj, H., Blake, B. & Wilhelmsen, L. (1977) 'Ability of spirometry, flow volume curves and the nitrogen closing volume test to detect smokers', *Scand. J. Resp. Dis.*, *58*, 80–96

Palmgren, B., Wahlen, R. & Wallander, B. (1973) 'Toxemia and cigarette smoking during pregnancy. Prospective consecutive investigation of 3,927 pregnancies', *Acta Obst. Gynecol. Scand.*, *52*, 183–5

Palmgren, B. & Wallander, B. (1971) 'Cigarettrokning och abort', *Konsekutiv prospectiv Undersokning av 4,312 Graviditeter, Lakartidningen*, *68* (22), 2611–16

Panayotopoulos, S., Gotsis, N., Papazoglou, N. & Concouris, L. (1974) 'Antigenic study of nicotiana tabacum and research on precipitins against tobacco antigens in the serum of smokers and non-smokers', *Allergologia et Immunopathologia*, *2*, 111–14

Pankow, D., Ponsold, W. & Fritz, H. (1974) 'Combined effects of carbon monoxide and ethanol on the effects of leucine amino-peptidase and glutamic-pyruvic transaminase in the plasma of rats', *Arch. Toxikol.*, *32*, 331–40

Parke, D.W. (1975) 'This doctor is firm: "I advise my patients not to smoke"', *Amer. Lung. Assoc. Bull.*, *61*, 7–9

Pascasio, F., Scassellati Sforzolini, G., Savino, A. & Conti, R. (1966) 'Catrame e nicotina nella porzione aspirata e nella porzione ambientale del fumo di vari tipi di sigarette', *Ann. della Sanita Pubblica*, *27*, 971–8

Pattee, H.E. (1969) 'Production of aflatoxins by Aspergillus flavus cultured on flue-cured tobacco', *Appl. Microbiol.*, *18*, 952–3

Pechstein, L.A. & Reynolds, W.R. (1937) 'Effect of tobacco smoke on growth and learning behavior of albino rat and its progeny', *J. Comparat. Psychol.*, *24*, 459–69

Penkala, S.J. & De Oliviera, G. (1975) 'The simultaneous analysis of carbon monoxide and suspended particulate matter produced by cigarette smoking', *Environ. Res.*, *9*, 99–114

Perdriel, G. (1975) 'Les affections psychosomatiques oculaires', *Entretiens de Bichat. Therapeutique*, *1*, 283–5

Perdriel, G., Lauthony, P. & Chevaleraud, J. (1975) 'Dyschromatopsies acquises reconnaissant une cause génerale ou toxique', Bull. des Soc. d'Ophthalmol. de France (special issue), 194–201

Perkin, G.D., Bowden, P. & Rose, F.C. (1975) 'Smoking and optic neuritis', *Postgrad. Med. J.*, *51*, 382–5

Perkin, G.D. & Rose, F.C. (1976) 'Uhtholff's syndrome', *Brit. J. Ophthalmol.*, *60*, 60–3

Perlman, H.H., Dannënberg, A.M. & Sokoloff, N. (1942) 'The excretion of nicotine in breast milk and urine from cigarette smoking. Its effect on lactation and the nursling', *J. Amer. Med. Assoc.*, *120*, 1003–9

Permutt, S. & Farhi, L. (1969) 'Tissue hypoxia and carbon monoxide' in A.B. Dubois (Chairman, ed.), *Effects of chronic exposure to low levels of carbon monoxide on human health, behavior and performance*, National Academy of Sciences, National Academy of Engineering, Washington, DC

Persson, P.H., Grennert, L., Gennser, G. & Kullander, S. (1978) 'A study of smoking and pregnancy with special reference to fetal growth', *Acta Obstetr. Gynecol. Scand. Suppl.*, *78*, 33–9

Peshkin, M.M. & Landay, L.H. (1939) 'Cutaneous reactions to tobacco antigen in allergic and non-allergic children with the direct and indirect (local passive transfer) methods of testing', *J. Allergy*, *10*, 241–5

Peterson, W.F., Morese, K.N. & Kaltreider, D.F. (1965) 'Smoking and prematurity. A preliminary report based on study of 7,740 Caucasians', *Obst. Gynecol.*, *26*, 775–9

Pettigrew, A.R. & Fell, G.S. (1972) 'Simplified colorimetric determination of

182   *References*

thiocyanate in biological fluids, and its application to investigation of the toxic amblyopias', *Clin. Chem.*, *18*, 996–1000
—— (1973) 'Microdiffusion method for estimation of cyanide in whole blood and its application to the study of conversion of cyanide to thiocyanate', *Clin. Chem.*, *19*, 466–71

Pimm, P., Shephard, R.J. & Silverman, F. (1978) 'Physiological effects of acute exposure to cigarette smoke', *Arch. Env. Health*, *33*, 201–13

Pipes, D.M. (1945) 'Allergy to tobacco smoke', *Ann. Allergy*, *28*, 277–82

Pirani, B.B.K. (1978) 'Smoking during pregnancy', *Obstetr. Gyn. Survey*, *33*, 1–13

Pirani, B.B.K. & MacGillivray, I. (1978) 'Smoking during pregnancy: its effects on maternal metabolism and fetoplacental function', *Amer. J. Obstetr. Gynecol.*, *52*, 257–63

Pitts, G.C. & Pace, N. (1947) 'The effect of blood carboxyhemoglobin concentration on hypoxia tolerance', *Amer. J. Physiol.*, *148*, 139–51

Pollard, M.R. & Brennan, J.T. (1978) 'Disease prevention and health promotion initiatives: some legal considerations', *Health Educ. Monogr.*, *6*, 211–22

Portheine, F. (1972) 'Das Sogennante passive Rauchen', *Rehabilitation*, *25*, 33–4

Potts, A.M. (1973) 'Tobacco amblyopia', *Survey of Ophthalmology*, *17*, 313–39

Power, G.G. & Longo, L.D. (1975) 'Fetal circulation times and their implications for tissue oxygenation', *Gynecol. Invest.*, *6*, 342–55

Quigley, M.E., Sheehan, K.L., Wilkes, M.M. & Yen, S.S.C. (1979) 'Effects of maternal smoking on circulating catecholamine levels and fetal heart rates', *Amer. J. Obstetr. Gynecol.*, *133*, 685–90

Radojicic, B. (1973) 'Odredivanje rodanida u mokraci u radnika izlozenih cijanidima', *Archiv za Higijenu Rada i Toksikologiju*, *24*, 227–32

Ramsey, J.M. (1972) 'Carbon monoxide, tissue hypoxia and sensory psychomotor response in hypoxemia', *Clin. Sci.*, *42*, 619–25

Rantakallio, P. (1969) 'Groups at risk in low birth weight infants and perinatal mortality. A prospective study of the biological characteristics and socioeconomic circumstances of mothers in 12,000 deliveries in North Finland 1966. A discriminant function analysis', *Acta Paed. Scand.* (Suppl. 193), 1–77
—— (1978a) 'The effect of maternal smoking on birth weight and the subsequent health of the child', *Early Hum. Dev.*, *2*, 371–82
—— (1978b) 'Relationship of maternal smoking to morbidity and mortality of the child up to the age of five', *Acta Paed. Scand.*, *67*, 621–31

Rantakallio, P., Krause, U. & Krause, K. (1979) 'The use of ophthalmological services during the preschool age, occular findings and family background', *J. Pediatr. Ophthalm. Strabismus*, *15*, 253–8

Raven, P.B., Drinkwater, B.L., Ruhling, R.O., Bolduan, N., Taguchi, S., Gliner, J. & Horvath, S.M. (1974) 'Effect of carbon monoxide and peroxyacetyl nitrate on man's maximal aerobic capacity', *J. Appl. Physiol.*, *36*, 288–93

Ravenholt, R.T. & Levinski, M.J. (1965) 'Smoking during pregnancy', *Lancet*, (*1*), 961

Ravenholt, R.T., Levinski, M.J., Nellist, D.J. & Takenaga, M. (1966) 'Effects of smoking upon reproduction', *Amer. J. Obstetr. Gyn.*, *96*, 267–81

Ray, A.M. & Rockwell, T.H. (1970) 'An exploratory study of automobile driving performance under the influence of low levels of carboxyhemoglobin', *Ann. N.Y. Acad. Sci.*, *174*, 396–407

Reece, W.O. & Ball, R.A. (1972) 'Inhaled cigarette smoke and treadmill-exercised dogs', *Arch. Env. Health*, *24*, 262–70

Regan, T.J., Frank, M.J., McGinty, J.F., Zobl, E., Hellems, H.K. & Bing, R.J.

(1961) 'Myocardial response to cigarette smoking in normal subjects and patients with coronary disease', *Circulation, 23*, 365-9

Reid, L. (1960) 'Chronic bronchitis and hypersecretion of mucus' in *Lectures on the Scientific Basis of Medicine, 8*, Butterworth Scientific Publications, London

Reintjes, M., Swierenga, J. & Bogaard, J.M. (1972) 'Effects of smoking one cigarette on airway resistance', *Scand. J. Resp. Dis., 53*, 129-34

Resnik, R., Brink, G.W. & Wilkes, M. (1979) 'Catecholamine-mediated reduction in uterine blood flow after nicotine infusion in the pregnant ewe', *J. Clin. Invest., 63*, 1113-36

Rhead, W.J. (1977) 'Smoking and SIDS', *Pediatrics, 59*, 719-92

Rickert, W.S. (1981) 'Tar nicotine figures on package not telling whole story, test show – Price Watch – M. Anderson', *Toronto Star*, 1 March 1981

Roach, S.A. (1973) 'Industrial ventilation' in R.S.F. Schilling (ed.), *Occupational health practice*, Butterworths, London, pp. 339-59

Robinson, J.C. & Forbes, W.F. (1975) 'The role of carbon monoxide in cigarette smoking. I. Carbon monoxide yield from cigarettes', *Arch. Environ. Health, 30*, 425-34

Rockwell, T.J. & Ray, A.M. (1967) 'Subacute carbon monoxide poisoning and driving performance: a selected review of the literature and discussion', *A report to the National Safety Council*, Chicago, Ill.

Rockwell, T.J. & Weir, F.W. (1975) *The interactive effects of carbon monoxide and alcohol on driving skills*, Ohio State University Research Foundation, RF Project 332, pp. 1-112

Rode, A., Ross, R. & Shephard, R.J. (1972) 'Smoking withdrawal program', *AMA Arch Env. Health, 24*, 27-36

Rode, A. & Shephard, R.J. (1971) 'The influence of cigarette smoking upon the work of breathing in near maximal exercise', *Med. Sci. Sports, 3*, 51-5

Rosen, F.L. (1954) 'Studies in tobacco allergy', *J. Med. Soc., New Jersey, 51*, 109-14

Rosen, F.L. & Levy, A. (1950) 'Bronchial asthma due to allergy to tobacco smoke in an infant', *J. Amer. Med. Assoc., 144*, 620-1

Rosenmann, R.H., Brand, R.J., Sholtz, R.I. & Jenkins, C.D. (1974) 'Relation of corneal arcus to cardiovascular risk factors and the incidence of coronary diseases', *New Engl. J. Med., 291*, 1322-4

Ross, J.C., Ley, G.D., Krumholz, R.A. & Rahbari, H. (1967) 'A technique for evaluation of gas mixing in the lung: studies in cigarette smokers and non-smokers', *Amer. Rev. Resp. Dis., 95*, 447-53

Rossmann, H. (1970) 'Vitamin B_{12} resorption bei der sogennanten Tabak-Amblyopie', *Dtsch. Med. Wochenschr., 95*, 419-20

Rottenstein, H., Peirce, G., Russ, E., Felder, O. & Montgomery, H. (1960) 'Influence of nicotine on the blood flow of resting skeletal muscle and of the digits in normal subjects', *Ann. N.Y. Acad. Sci., 90*, 102-13

Rowell, P.P. & Sastry, B.V.R. (1977) 'Human placental cholinergic system: effects of cholinergic blockade on amino acid uptake in isolated placental villi', *Fed. Proc., 36*, 981

—— (1978) 'The influence of cholinergic blockade on the uptake of amino-isobutyric acid by isolated human placental villi', *Toxicol. Appl. Pharmacol., 45*, 79-93

Royal College of Physicians (London) (1962) *Smoking and Health*, Pitman Medical Publishing, London

—— (1977) *Smoking or health – the third report from the Royal College of Physicians, London*, Pitman, London

Rummel, R.M., Crawford, M. & Bruce, P. (1975) 'The physiological effects of

inhaling exhaled cigarette smoke in relation to attitude of the non-smoker',
J. Sch. Health, *45*, 524-9

Rummo, N. & Sarlanis, K. (1974) 'The effect of carbon monoxide on several
measures of vigilance in a simulated driving task', *J. Safety Res.*, *6*, 126-30

Rush, D. (1974) 'Examination of the relationship between birth weight, cigarette
smoking during pregnancy and maternal weight gain', *J. Obst. Gynaecol. Brit.
Commonw.*, *81*, 746-52

—— (1979) 'Effects of smoking on pregnancy and newborn infants', *Amer. J.
Obstetr. Gynecol.*, *135*, 281-2

Russell, C.S., Taylor, R. & Law, C.E. (1968) 'Smoking in pregnancy, maternal
blood pressure, pregnancy outcome, baby weight and growth and other
related factors. A prospective study', *Brit. J. Prev. Soc. Med.*, *22*, 119-26

Russell, C.S., Taylor, R. & Maddison, R.N. (1966) 'Some effects of smoking in
pregnancy', *J. Obstetr. Gynaecol. Brit. Commonw.*, *73*, 742-6

Russell, M.A.H. (1980) 'The case for medium-nicotine, low tar, low carbon
monoxide cigarettes' in G.B. Gori & F.G. Bock (eds.), *Banbury Report 3 –
A safe cigarette*, Cold Spring Harbor Laboratory, Cold Spring Harbor, NY,
pp. 297-310

Russell, M.A.H., Cole, P.V. & Brown, E. (1973) 'Absorption by non-smokers of
carbon monoxide from room air polluted by tobacco smoke', *Lancet*, *(i)*
(7803), 576-9

Russell, M.A.H. & Feyerabend, C. (1975) 'Blood and urinary nicotine in non-
smokers', *Lancet*, *(i)* (7900), 179-81

Russell, M.A.H., Sutton, S.R., Feyerabend, C., Cole, P.V. & Saloojee, Y. (1977)
'Nicotine chewing gum as a substitute for smoking', *Brit. Med. J.*, *(i)*, 1060-3

Said, G. & Zalokar, J. (1978) 'Incidence des affections respiratoires supérieures
chez les enfants des fumeurs', *Ann. d'Oto-Laryngol. Chir. Cervico-Fac.*, *95*,
236-40

Sanford, M., Gieser, M.T. & Czesak, K. (1978) *Report on the impact of the
Berkeley smoking pollution control act of 1977* (Ordinance No. 4983-N),
Wright Institute, Berkeley, Calif., 1 June 1978

Savel, H. (1970) 'Clinical hypersensitivity to cigarette smoke', *Arch. Env. Health*,
21, 146-8

Savel, L.E. & Roth, E. (1962) 'Effects of smoking in pregnancy. A continuing
retrospective study', *Obstetr. Gynecol.*, *20*, 313-16

Saxton, D.W. (1978) 'The behavior of infants whose mothers smoke in pregnancy',
Early Hum. Dev., *2*, 363-9

Scassellati Sforzolini, G. & Savino, A. (1968) 'Valutazione di un indice rapido di
contaminazione ambientale da fumo di sigaretta, in relazione alla
composizione della gassosa del fumo', *Rivista Ital. D'Igiene*, *28*, 43-55

Schilling, R.S.F., Letai, A.D., Hui, S.L., Beck, G.J., Schoenberg, J.B. &
Bouhuys, A. (1977) 'Lung function, respiratory disease and smoking in
families', *Amer. J. Epidemiol.*, *106*, 274-83

Schlede, E. & Merker, H.J. (1972) 'Effect of benzo (α) pyrene treatment on the
benzo (α) pyrene hydroxylase activity in maternal liver, placenta and fetus
of the rat during Day 13 to Day 18 of gestation', *Naunyn Schmied. Arch.
Pharmacol.*, *272*, 89-100

Schlotzhauer, W.S., Higman, E.B. & Schmeltz, I. (1972) 'Pyrolysis of tobacco
extracts' in I. Schmeltz (ed.), *The chemistry of tobacco and tobacco smoke*,
Plenum Press, New York, pp. 65-76

Schmeltz, I., Abidi, S., & Hoffmann, D. (1977) 'Tumorigenic agents in unburned
processed tobacco: N-nitrosodiethanolamine and 1,1-dimethylhydrazine',
Cancer Letters, *2* (3), 125-32

Schmeltz, I., Brunnemann, K.D., Hoffmann, D. & Cornell, A. (1976) 'On the chemistry of cigar smoke: comparisons between experimental little and large cigars', *Beitr. zur Tabakforsch.*, *8*, 367–77

Schmeltz, I. & Hoffmann, D. (1977) 'Nitrogen-containing compounds in tobacco and tobacco smoke', *Chem. Rev.*, *77*, 295–311

Schmidt, B. (1970) 'Einfluss des Zigarettenrauchens auf das EOG', *Klin. Monatsblatter für Augenheilkunde*, *156*, 523–31

Schoeneck, F.J. (1941) 'Cigarette smoking in pregnancy', *New York State J. Med.*, *41*, 1945–8

Schorah, C.J., Zemroch, P.J., Sheppard, S. & Smithells, R.W. (1978) 'Leucocyte ascorbic acid and pregnancy', *Brit. J. Nutr.*, *39*, 139–49

Schrauzer, G.N., Rhead, W.J. & Saitzstee, S.L. (1975) 'Sudden infant death syndrome. Plasma vitamin E levels and dietary factors', *Ann. Clin. Lab. Sci.*, *5*, 31–7

Schur, M.O. & Rickards, J.C. (1957) *Tobacco Sci.*, *1*, 13–20

——— (1960) 'Design of low yield cigarettes', *Tobacco Sci.*, *4*, 69–77

Schwartz, D., Goujard, J., Kaminski, M. & Rumeau-Rouquette, C. (1972) 'Smoking and pregnancy. Results of a prospective study of 6,989 women', *Rev. Europ. Ét. Clin. Biol.*, *17*, 867–79

Schwartz, J. (1977) 'Anti-smoking movement – Part I. Program Gains Momentum', *Health Sciences J.*, *5* (1), 8

Scoughton, C.R. & Heimstra, N.W. (1973) 'The effects of smoking on peripheral movement detection', unpublished report, Dept. of Psychology, University of S. Dakota, Vermilion, S. Dakota, pp. 1–45

Sebben, J., Pimm, P. & Shephard, R.J. (1977) 'Cigarette smoke in enclosed public facilities', *Arch. Env. Health*, *32*, 53–8

Seiff, H.E. (1973) *Carbon monoxide as an indicator of cigarette-caused pollution levels in intercity buses*, US Dept. of Transportation, Federal Highway Administration, Beareau of Motor Carrier Safety, pp. 1–11

Sem, G.J. & Tsurubayashi, K. (1975) 'A new mass sensor for respirable dust measurement', *Amer. Industr. Hyg. Assoc. J.*, *36*, 791–800

Seppänen, A. (1977a) 'Smoking in closed space and its effect on carboxyhaemoglobin saturation of smoking and non-smoking subjects', *Ann. Clin. Res.*, *9*, 281–3

——— (1977b) 'Physical work capacity in relation to carbon monoxide inhalation and tobacco smoking', *Ann. Clin. Res.*, *9*, 269–74

Shephard, R.J. (1966) 'The oxygen cost of breathing during vigorous exercise', *Quart. J. Exp. Physiol.*, *51*, 336–50

——— (1976) 'Exercise and training in chronic obstructive lung disease', *Exercise Sports Sci. Rev.*, *5*, 263–96

——— (1977) *Endurance Fitness*, 2nd edn, Univ. of Toronto Press, Toronto

——— (1978a) *Human physiological work capacity*, Cambridge University Press, London

——— (1978b) 'Cigarette smoking and reactions to air pollutants', *Canad. Med. Assoc. J.*, *118*, 379–83, 392

——— (1981a) *Carbon monoxide – an air quality criterion for the working environment*, Health & Welfare, Canada, Ottawa

——— (1981b) *Air quality criteria for carbon monoxide*, Health & Welfare, Canada, Ottawa

Shephard, R.J., Carey, G.C.R. & Phair, J.J. (1958) 'Critical evaluation of a filter-strip smoke sampler used in domestic premises', *AMA Arch. Industr. Health*, *17*, 236–52

Shephard, R.J., Collins, R. & Silverman, F. (1979a) 'Responses of exercising subjects to acute "passive" cigarette smoke exposure', *Environ. Res.*, *19*, 279–91

186   *References*

——— (1979b) '"Passive" exposure of asthmatic subjects to cigarette smoke', *Environ. Res.*, *20*, 392–402

Shephard, R.J. & LaBarre, R. (1976) *Attitudes to smoking and cigarette smoke. The Toronto Survey, 1976*, York-Toronto Respiratory Disease Association, Willowdale, Ont.

——— (1978) 'Attitudes of the public towards cigarette smoke in public places', *Canad. J. Publ. Health*, *69*, 302–10

Shephard, R.J. & Lorimer, J. (in press) 'Attitudes towards the hazards of smoking: the influence of pregnancy', *Ind. J. Chest Dis.*

Shephard, R.J., Ponsford, E., Basu, P.K. & LaBarre, R. (1978a) *Reactions to passive cigarette smoke exposure. The 1977 Toronto Survey*, York-Toronto Respiratory Disease Association, Willowdale, Ont.

——— (1978b) 'Effects of cigarette smoking on intraocular pressure and vision', *Brit. J. Ophthalmol.*, *62*, 682–7

——— (1979c) 'Effect of cigarette smoke on the eyes and airway', *Int. Arch. Occup. Environ. Health*, *43*, 135–44

Shepherd, J.T. (1951) 'Effect of cigarette smoking on blood flow through the hand', *Brit. Med. J.*, (*ii*), 1007–10

Shimp, D.M., Blumrosen, A.W. & Finifter, S.B. (1976) *How to protect your health at work*, Environmental Improvement Associates, Salem, NJ

Shy, C.M., Creason, J.P., Pearlman, M.E., McClain, K.E. & Benson, F.B. (1970) 'The Chattanooga school children study. Effects of community exposure to nitrogen dioxide. II. Incidence of acute respiratory illness', *J. Air. Poll. Contr. Assoc.*, *20*, 582–8

Silverman, J.T. (1977) 'Maternal smoking and birthweight', *Amer. J. Epidemiol.*, *105*, 513–21

Simpson, W.J. (1957) 'A preliminary report on cigarette smoking and the incidence of prematurity', *Amer. J. Obstetr. Gynecol.*, *73*, 808–15

Sjöstrand, T. (1948) 'A method for the determination of carboxyhemoglobin concentrations by analysis of alveolar air', *Acta Physiol. Scand.*, *16*, 201–10

Slavin, R.G. & Hertz, M. (1975) 'Indoor air pollution', paper presented to Amer. Acad. Allergy, San Diego, Calif., 15–19 February 1975

Smith, E., McMillan, E. & Mack, L. (1935) 'Factors influencing the lethal action of illuminating gas', *J. Industr. Hyg.*, *17*, 18–20

Sodano, A. (1934) 'Ricerche sperimentali sull influenza della nicotina sulla funzione genitale della donna', *Arch. Ostetr. Ginecol.*, *1*, 559–69

Sontag, L.W. & Wallace, R.F. (1935) 'The effect of cigaret smoking during pregnancy upon the fetal heart rate', *Amer. J. Obstetr. Gyn.*, *29*, 77–83

South African Dept. of Health (1977) 'The health hazards of smoking', *S. Afr. Med. J.*, *52*, 419–20

Soyka, F. & Edmonds, A. (1977) *The ion effect*, E.P. Dutton, New York

Spears, A.W., Bell, J.H. & Saunders, A.O. (1965) Cited by E.L. Wynder & Hoffmann, D. (1967). 19th Tobacco Chemists Research Conference, Lexington, Kentucky, pp. 29–31

Speer, F. (1968) 'Tobacco and the non-smoker. A study of subjective symptoms', *Arch. Environ. Health*, *16*, 443–6

——— (1971) 'Passenger smoking effects on bus driver' (letter), *Arch. Env. Health*, *22*, 512

Spira, A., Phillipe, E., Spira, N., Dreyfus, J. & Schwartz, D. (1977) 'Smoking during pregnancy and placental pathology', *Biomed.*, *27*, 266–70

Srch, M. (1967) 'Ueber die Bedeutung des Kohlenoxyds beim Zigarettenrauchen im Personenkraftwageninnern', *Dtsch. Z. f. die Ges. Gerichtliche Med.*, *60*, 80–9

Stahle, I. & Tibbling, L. (1978) 'Tobaksallergi hos Patienter med Asthma bronchiale', *Lakartidningen*, 75, 1711–13

Stedman, R.L. (1968) 'The chemical composition of tobacco and tobacco smoke', *Chem. Rev.*, 68, 153–207

Steele, R. & Langworth, J.T. (1966) 'The relationship of antenatal and postnatal factors to sudden unexpected death in infancy', *Canad. Med. Assoc. J.*, 94, 1165–71

Steinberg, R.A. & Jeffrey, R.N. (1956) 'Effect of micronutrient deficiencies on nicotine formation by tobacco in water culture', *Plant Physiol.*, 31, 377–82

Sterling, G.M. (1967) 'Mechanism of bronchoconstriction caused by cigarette smoking', *Brit. Med. J.*, (ii), 275–6

Stewart, R.D., Baretta, E.D., Platte, L.R., Stewart, E.B., Kalbfleisch, J.H., Yserloo, B. Van & Rimm, A.A. (1974) 'Carboxyhemoglobin levels in American blood donors', *J. Amer. Med. Assoc.*, 229, 1187–95

Stewart, R.D., Peterson, J.E., Baretta, E.D., Bachand, M.T., Hosko, M.J. & Herrmann, A.A. (1970) 'Experimental human exposure to carbon monoxide', *Arch. Env. Health*, 21, 154–64

Stock, S. (1980) 'The perils of second-hand smoking', *New Scientist*, 2 (October 1980), 10–13

Stone, H. (1963) 'Influence of temperature on olfactory sensitivity', *J. Appl. Physiol.*, 18, 746–51

Sugimura, T., Sato, S., Nagao, M., Yahagi, T., Matsushima, T., Seino, Y., Takeuchi, M. & Kawachi, T. (1976) 'Over-lapping of carcinogens and mutagens' in P.N. Magee, S. Takayama, T. Sugimura & T. Matsushima (eds.), *Fundamentals in cancer prevention*, University Park Press, Baltimore

Sulzberger, M.B. (1933) 'Studies in tobacco hypersensitivity. I. A comparison between reactions to nicotine and to denicotinized tobacco extract', *J. Immunol.*, 24, 85–91

Surgeon General, (1979) *Smoking and health*, Washington DC, DHEW Publication PHS 79–50066

———— (1980) *The health consequences of smoking for women*, US Govt. Printing Office, Washington, DC

———— (1981) *The health consequences of smoking. The changing cigarette*, US Dept. of Health and Human Services, Public Health Service, 81–50156

Suzuki, K., Horiguchi, T., Comas-Urrutia, A.C., Mueller-Heubach, E., Morishima, H.O. & Adamsons, J. (1971) 'Pharmacologic effects of nicotine upon the fetus and mother in the pregnant Rhesus monkey', *Amer. J. Obstetr. Gynecol.*, 111, 1092–101

Szadkowski, D., Harke, H.P. & Angerer, J. (1976) 'Kohlenmonoxidbelastung durch Passivrauchen in Bueroraumen', *Innere Medizin*, 3, 310–13

Szadkowski, E., Schultze, H., Schaller, H.H. & Lehnert, G. (1969) Zur ökologischen Bedeutung des Schwermetallgehaltes von Zigaretten, Blei, Cadmium und Nickelanalysen des Tabaks sowie der Gas- und Partikelphase', *Arch. Hyg. Bakteriol.*, 153, 1–8

Tager, I.B., Weiss, S.T., Rosner, B. & Speizer, F.E. (1979) 'Effect of parental cigarette smoking on the pulmonary function of children', *Amer. J. Epidemiol.*, 110, 15–26

Tanaka, M. (1965) 'Studies on the etiological mechanism of fetal developmental disorders caused by maternal smoking during pregnancy', *Nippon Sanka-Fujinka Gakkai Zasshi*, 17, 1107–14

Taylor, G. (1974) 'Tobacco smoke allergy – does it exist?' in R. Rylander (ed.), *Environmental Tobacco Smoke. Effects on the Non-Smoker*, Scand. J. Resp. Dis. Suppl., 95, pp. 50–5

Thayer, W.W. (1981) 'Tobacco smoke dilution recommendations for satisfactory ventilation', *A.S.H.R.A.W. log 2086*, 30 April 1981, 1–24 + tables

Theodore, J. (1973) 'Angina pectoris and carbon monoxide' (letter), *Ann. Int. Med.*, *78*, 455

Theodore, J., O'Donnell, R.D. & Back, K.C. (1971) 'Toxicological evaluation of carbon monoxide in humans and other mammalian species', *J. Occup. Med.*, *13*, 242–55

Thienes, C.H., Lombard, C.F., Fielding, F.J., Lesser, A.J. & Ellenhorn, M.J. (1946) 'Alterations in reproductive functions of white rats associated with daily exposure to nicotine', *J. Pharmacol. Expt. Therap.*, *87*, 1–10

Thomas, C.B., Bateman, J.L. & Lindberg, E.F. (1956) 'Observations on the individual effects of smoking on the blood pressure, heart rate, stroke volume and cardiac output of healthy young adults', *Ann. Int. Med.*, *44*, 874–92

Thompson, W.B. (1933) 'Nicotine in breast milk', *Amer. J. Obstetr. Gyn.*, *26*, 662–7

Thomsen, H.K. & Kjeldsen, K. (1974) 'Threshold limit for carbon-monoxide-induced myocardial damage. An electron microscopic study in rabbits', *Arch. Environ. Health*, *29*, 73–8

Thomson, M.L. & Pavia, D. (1973) 'Long-term tobacco smoking and muco-ciliary clearance', *A.M.A. Arch. Env. Health*, *26*, 86–90

Tillmanns, H., Sarma, I.S.M., Seeler, K., *et al.* (1975) 'Lipid metabolism in perfused human coronary arteries and saphenous veins' in G. Schettler & A. Weizel (eds.), *Atherosclerosis Vol. 3*, Springer Verlag, New York, pp. 118–25

Tjalve, H., Hansson, E. & Schmiterlow, C.G. (1968) 'Passage of ^{14}C nicotine and its metabolites into mice foetuses and placentae', *Acta Pharmacol. Toxicol.*, *26*, 539–55

Tobacco (1977) '8-point antismoking drive launched in U.K.', *Tobacco*, *129*, 19–20

Touey, G.P. & Mumpower, R.C. (1957) *Tobacco Sci.*, *1*, 33–7

Trasoff, A., Blumstein, G. & Marks, M. (1936) 'The immunologic aspect of tobacco in thromboangiitis obliterans and coronary artery disease', *J. Allergy*, *7*, 250–3

Truhaut, R., de Clercq, M. & Loisillier, F. (1964) 'Sur les toxicités aigue et chronique de la cotinine, et sur son effet cancérigène chez le rat', *Pathol. Biol.*, *12*, 39–49

Tso, T.C. (1975) 'Tobacco and tobacco smoke', in W.F. Childers & G.M. Russo (eds.), *Nightshades and health*, Somerset Press, Somerville, NJ, pp. 93–121

——— (1977) *Physiology and biochemistry of tobacco plants*, Dowden, Hutchinson & Ross, Stroudsberg, Pa.

Tso, T.C. & Gori, G.B. (1972) 'Effect of tobacco characteristics on cigarette smoke composition' in I. Schmeltz (ed.), *The chemistry of tobacco and tobacco smoke*, Plenum Press, New York, pp. 51–63

Tso, T.C., Lowe, R. & Dejong, D.W. (1975) 'Homogenized leaf curing. I. Theoretical basis and some preliminary results', *Beitr. Zur Tabakforsch.*, *7*, 190–4

Underwood, P., Hester, L.L., Laffitte, T. & Gregg, K.V. (1965) 'The relationship of smoking to the outcome of pregnancy', *Amer. J. Obst. Gynecol.*, *91*, 270–6

Underwood, P.B., Kesler, K.F., O'Lane, J.M., Callagan, D.A. (1967) 'Parental smoking empirically related to pregnancy outcome', *Obstetr. Gynecol.*, *29*, 1–8

US House of Representative (1978) 'Effect of smoking on non-smokers', Hearing before the subcommittee on Tobacco of the Committee on Agriculture, Serial 95–000, 7 August 1978, pp. 1–345

US National Clearing House for Smoking and Health (1976) *Adult use of tobacco, 1975*, US Dept. of Health, Education and Welfare, Public Health Service, June 1976

US Surgeon General (1972) *The health consequences of smoking*, US Dept. of Health, Education & Welfare, Arlington, Va.

Van den Berg, B.J. (1977) 'Epidemiologic observations of prematurity: effects of tobacco, coffee and alcohol' in D.M. Reed & F.J. Stanley (eds.), *The epidemiology of prematurity*, Urban & Schwarzenburg, Baltimore, pp. 157–71

Vanderslice, J. (1976) 'State laws on smoking in public places', *Amer. Lung. Assoc. Bull.*, *62*, 8–10

Viczian, M. (1969) 'Results of spermatozoa studies in cigarette smokers', *Z. f. Haut und Geschlechts-Krankheiten*, *44*, 183–7

Vogel, J.A. & Gleser, M.A. (1972) 'Effect of carbon monoxide on oxygen transport during exercise', *J. Appl. Physiol.*, *32*, 234–9

Vogt, T.M., Selvin, S., Widdowson, G. & Hulley, S.B. (1977) 'Expired air carbon monoxide and serum thiocyanate as objective measures of cigarette exposure', *Amer. J. Publ. Health*, *67*, 545–9

Vosburgh, J.A. & Vosburgh, L. (1977) 'Tobacco smoking in public places', *Env. Policy & Law*, *3*, 34–6

Waheed, M.A. & Basu, P.K. (1970) 'The effect of air pollutants on the eye. I. The effect of an organic extract on the conjunctival goblet cells', *Canad. J. Ophthalmol.*, *5*, 226–30

Wahl, F. (1899) 'Veber den Gehalt des Tabakrauches an Kohlenoxyd. Pflüg.', *Archiv. für die ges. Physiol.*, *88*, 262–85

Waite, C.L. (1978) Letter to the editor, *New Engl. J. Med.*, *299*, 897

Wakeham, H. (1972) 'Recent trends in tobacco and tobacco smoke research' in I. Schmeltz (ed.), *The chemistry of tobacco and tobacco smoke*, Plenum Press, New York, pp. 1–20

——— (1976) 'Sales-weighted average "tar" and nicotine deliveries of U.S. cigarettes from 1957 to present' in E.L. Wynder & S.S. Hecht (eds.), *Lung Cancer. A series of workshops on the biology of human cancer. Rept. 3*, Internat. Union Against Cancer, Geneva, Tech. Rept. Series 25, pp. 151–2

Wakeham, H.R.R. (1977) 'Environmental carbon monoxide from cigarette smoke – a critique', *Prev. Medicine*, *6*, 526–34

Waltz, P. & Hauserman, M. (1960) 'Investigations on the methodology of smoking. III. Approximate procedures for the determination of the puff volume from data from observations of smokers', *Mitt. Gebiete Lebensm. Hyg.*, *51*, 325–38

Wanner, A., Hirsch, J.A., Greeneltch, E. & Swenson, W. (1973) 'Tracheal mucous velocity after chronic exposure to cigarette smoke', *Arch. Env. Health*, *27*, 370–2

Watanabe, R., McIlrath, W.J., Skok, J., Chorney, W. & Wender, S.H. (1961) 'Accumulation of scopoletin in boron-deficient tobacco leaves', *Arch. Biochem. Biophys.*, *94*, 241–3

Weber, A., Fischer, T., Sancin, E. & Grandjean, E. (1976a) 'La pollution de l'air par la fumée de cigarettes; effets physiologiques et irritations', *Soz. und Praev. Med.*, *21*, 130–2

Weber, A., Jermini, C. & Grandjean, E. (1976b) 'Irritating effects on man of air pollution due to cigarette smoke', *Amer. J. Publ. Health*, *66*, 672–6

Weber-Tschoop, A., Fischer, T. & Grandjean, E. (1977a) 'Reizwirkungen des Formaldehyds (HCHO) auf den Menschen', *Int. Arch. Occup. Health*, *39*, 207–18

Weber-Tschoop, A., Fischer, T., Gierer, R. & Grandjean, E. (1977b) 'Experimentelle Reizwirkungen von Akrolein auf den Menschen', *Zeitschr. für Arbeitsmedizin*, *40 (2), 117–30*

Weber-Tschoop, A., Fischer, T. & Grandjean, E. (1976a) 'Objectiv und subjectiv physiologischen Wirkungen des Passivrauchens', *Int. Arch. Occup. Env. Health*,

37, 277–88

Weber-Tschoop, A., Jermini, C. & Grandjean, E. (1976b) 'Luftverunreinigung und Belaestigung durch Zigarettenrauch', *Soz. und Praev-Med.*, *21*, 101–6

Weir, F.W., Johnson, D.F., Anglen, D.M., Rockwell, T.H., Neuhardt, J.B., Harshman, D.J. & Balasubramanian, K.N. (1975) *The interactive effects of carbon monoxide and alcohol on driving skills*, Ohio State University Report, Columbus, Ohio, January 1975, pp. 1–112

Weir, F.W., Mehta, M.M., Johnson, D.F., Anglen, D.M., Rockwell, T.H., Attwood, D.A., Herrin, G.D. & Safford, R.R. (1973) *An investigation of the effects of carbon monoxide on humans in the driving task*, Ohio State University Research Fdn., January 1973

Welch, R.M., Gommi, B., Alvares, A.P., Conney, A.H. (1972) 'Effect of enzyme induction on the metabolism of benzo (α) pyrene and 3 methyl-4-monomethyl aminoazobenzene in the pregnant and fetal rat', *Cancer Res.*, *32*, 973–8

Welch, R.M., Harrison, Y.E., Conney, A.H., Poppers, P.J. & Finster, M. (1968) 'Cigarette smoking: stimulatory effect on metabolism of 3,4 benzpyrene by enzymes in human placenta', *Science*, *160*, 541–2

Westcott, F.H. & Wright, I.S. (1938) 'Tobacco allergy and thromboangiitis obliterans', *J. Allergy*, *9*, 555–64

Weybrew, J.A., Woltz, W.G. & Long, R.C. (1972) 'Projected changes in the composition of Bright (flue-cured) tobacco' in I. Schmeltz (ed.), *The chemistry of tobacco and tobacco smoke*, Plenum Press, New York, pp. 35–49

White, J.R. & Froeb, H.F. (1980) 'Small airways dysfunction in non-smokers chronically exposed to tobacco smoke', *New Engl. J. Med.*, *302*, 720–3

Williamson, J.T. & Allman, D.R. (1964) 'Effect of cigaret filter on the components of the vapor phase. Analysis of successive smoke puffs', *Beitr. Tabakforsch.*, *2*, 263–9

Williamson, J.T., Graham, J.F. & Allman, D.R. (1965) 'The modification of cigarette smoke by filter tips', *Beitr. Tabakforsch.*, *3*, 233–42

Willson, J.R. (1942) 'The effect of nicotine on lactation in white mice', *Amer. J. Obstetr. Gynecol.*, *43*, 839–44

Wilson, E.W. (1972) 'The effect of smoking in pregnancy on the placental coefficient', *New Z. Med. J.*, *74*, 384–5

Wilson, J., Linnell, J.C. & Matthews, D.M. (1971) 'Plasma cobalmins in neuro-ophthalmological disease', *Lancet*, (i), 259–61

Wilson, R.H., Meador, R.S., Jay, B.E. & Higgins, E. (1960) 'The pulmonary pathologic physiology of persons who smoke cigarettes', *New Engl. J. Med.*, *262*, 956–61

Wilson, W.S., Duncan, A.J. & Jay, J.L. (1975) 'Effect of benzalkonium chloride on the stability of the pre-corneal tear film in rabbit and man', *Brit. J. Ophthalmol.*, *59*, 667–9

Wingerd, J., Christianson, R., Lovitt, W.V. & Schoen, E.J. (1976) 'Placental ratio in white and black women, relation to smoking and anemia', *Amer. J. Obstetr. Gynecol.*, *124*, 671–5

Wingerd, J. & Schoen, E.J. (1974) 'Factors influencing length at birth and height at five years', *Pediatrics*, *53*, 737–41

Wingerd, J. & Sponzilli, E.E. (1977) 'Concentrations of serum protein fractions in white women: effects of age, weight, smoking, tonsillectomy and other factors', *Clin. Chem.*, *23*, 1310–17

World Health Organization (1960) *Constitution of the World Health Organization*, World Health Organization, Geneva

——— (1976) 'Legislative action to combat smoking around the world', *Int. Digest Health Legisl.*, *27*, 494–517

——— (1979) *Environmental health criteria 13. Carbon monoxide*, WHO, Geneva

Wright, G.R., Randell, P. & Shephard, R.J. (1973) 'Carbon monoxide and driving skills', *Arch. Environ. Health*, *27*, 349–54

Wright, G.R. & Shephard, R.J. (1978) 'Carbon monoxide exposure and auditory duration discrimination', *Arch. Environ. Health*, *33*, 226–35

Wynder, E.L. & Hoffmann, D. (1967) *Tobacco and tobacco smoke*, Academic Press, New York

Yabroff, I., Myers, E., Fend, V., David, N., Robertson, M., Wright, R. & Braun, R. (1974) *The role of atmospheric carbon monxide in vehicle accidents*, Standard Research Institute – Report on Contract CRC—APRAC Project CAPM 12-69, pp. 1–92

Yankelovich, Skelly & White, Inc. (1977) *A study of cigarette smoking among teen-age girls and young women. Summary of the findings*, National Cancer Inst., Washington, DC, DHEW (NIH) Publication 77, 1203

Yeates, D.B., Aspin, N., Levison, H., Jones, M.T. & Bryan, A.C. (1975) 'Mucociliary tracheal transport rates in man', *J. Appl. Physiol.*, *39*, 487–95

Yerushalmy, J. (1964) 'Mother's cigarette smoking and survival of infant', *Amer. J. Obstetr. Gynecol.*, *88*, 505–18

—— (1965) 'Cigarette smoking and infant survival', *Amer. J. Obstetr. Gynecol.*, *91*, 881–3

—— (1972) 'Infants with low birth weight born before their mothers started to smoke cigarettes', *Amer. J. Obstetr. Gynecol.*, *112*, 277–84

Yeung, D.L. (1976) 'Relationships between cigarette smoking, oral contraceptives and plasma vitamins A, E, C and plasma triglycerides and cholesterol', *Amer. J. Clin. Nutr.*, *29*, 1216–21

Yoshinaga, K., Rice, C., Krenn, J. & Pilot, R.L. (1979) 'Effects of nicotine on early pregnancy in the rat', *Biol. Reprod.*, *20*, 294–303

Young, S.H. & Stone, H.L. (1976) 'Effect of a reduction in arterial oxygen content (carbon monoxide) on coronary flow', *Aviat. Space Environ. Med.*, *47*, 142–6

Younoszai, M.K., Kacic, A. & Haworth, J.C. (1968) 'Cigarette smoking during pregnancy: the effect upon the haematocrit and acid-base balance of the newborn infant', *Canad. Med. Assoc. J.*, *99*, 197–200

Zabriskie, J.E. (1963) 'Effect of cigarette smoking during pregnancy', *Obstetr. Gynecol.*, *21*, 405–11

Zorn, H. (1972) 'The partial oxygen pressure in the brain and liver at subtoxic concentrations of carbon monoxide', *Staub-Reinhalt Luft*, *32*, 24–9

Zuskin, E., Mitchell, C.A. & Bouhuys, A. (1974) 'Interaction between effects of beta blockade and cigarette smoke on airways', *J. Appl. Physiol.*, *36*, 449–52

Zussman, B.M. (1970) 'Tobacco sensitivity in the allergic patient', *Ann. Allergy*, *28*, 371–7

—— (1974) 'Tobacco sensitivity in the allergic population', *J. Asthma Res.*, *11*, 159–68

INDEX

W. SUSSEX INSTITUTE
OF
HIGHER EDUCATION
LIBRARY